Lynch Syndrome

Naohiro Tomita
Editor

Lynch Syndrome

Molecular Mechanism and Current Clinical Practice

Springer

Editor
Naohiro Tomita
Specially Appointed Adviser
Cancer Treatment Center
Toyonaka Municipal Hospital
Osaka
Japan

Professor Emeritus
Division of Lower GI Surgery
Department of Surgery
Hyogo College of Medicine
Hyogo
Japan

ISBN 978-981-15-6893-0 ISBN 978-981-15-6891-6 (eBook)
https://doi.org/10.1007/978-981-15-6891-6

This Springer imprint is published by the registered company Springer Nature Singapore Pte Ltd.
The registered company address is: 152 Beach Road, #21-01/04 Gateway East, Singapore 189721, Singapore

Preface

Lynch syndrome (LS) is one of the most common hereditary cancer syndromes, which has specific clinical features such as early-onset cancer, multiple colorectal cancer, and extra-colonic cancer occurrence in various organs, including the endometrium, stomach, small intestine, urinary tract, hepatobiliary tract, and ovaries.

The history of LS commenced with a report published in 1913 by a dedicated pathologist Prof. Aldred S. Warthin at the University of Michigan, who had documented three families predisposed to multiple cancer involvement with suggestive autosomal dominant inheritance [1]. This syndrome was further investigated by Prof. Henry T. Lynch in 1966 [2], and the concept of "cancer family syndrome" gradually expanded worldwide.

The molecular mechanisms underlying the carcinogenesis of this syndrome have been investigated by many researchers, and finally, genes related to the mismatch repair (MMR) system during DNA replication were found to be the cause of this disease during the 1990s.

Four mismatch repair genes—*MSH2*, *MLH1*, *MSH6*, and *PMS2*—which are responsible for maintaining the genome fidelity by repairing base mismatches during DNA replication and a related gene, *EPCAM*, have been identified as causative genes for LS.

During the aforementioned stream of research in this field, the nomenclature of this syndrome has changed. It was once referred to as hereditary non-polyposis colorectal cancer (HNPCC); however, this nomenclature has been considered inappropriate because of this syndrome's nature with cancer occurrence in multiple organs other than the colorectum. The terminology "Lynch syndrome" was then defined as a hereditary cancer syndrome with autosomal dominant inheritance due to germline defects in the MMR system and is now used widely in general.

Clinical diagnostic criteria, including the Amsterdam criteria followed by the Amsterdam criteria II, have been developed and used for the clinical diagnosis of this syndrome. However, these criteria for LS diagnosis have major limitations. It has been reported that half of all LS cases may be missed by screening patients with colorectal cancer using the Amsterdam criteria [3]. These previously proposed criteria, together with the Bethesda guidelines, are not diagnostic criteria, but just one of the initial screening tools for LS. Furthermore, currently, universal screening that does not depend on these history-taking-based criteria has been proposed, and its clinical usefulness has been investigated in terms of various aspects.

Several guidelines for this hereditary disorder have been published thus far worldwide. In Japan, the guideline for hereditary colorectal cancer was published first in 2012 and was revised in 2016 [4]. Importantly, this revised version of the guideline was immediately translated into English and published [5]. Currently, it is under further complete revision, and the revised version of the Japanese guideline is scheduled to be published in July this year. Soon afterward, its English version will also be published.

Meanwhile, we are currently in an era of "genomic medicine," as is widely known. In particular, in the field of cancer, "cancer genomic medicine" is the mainstream focus, not only for diagnosis but also for the treatment of various cancers. Cancer gene panel examinations utilizing next-generation sequencing offer us the chance to choose appropriate drugs that possibly work directly against molecules associated with somatic disorders in cancer cells. However, during these examinations, some germline variants might be detected unexpectedly as so-called secondary findings. Importantly, these may indicate that an individual harbors a hereditary cancer syndrome disease with a germline genetic disorder.

In Japan, and probably also in other countries, few patients with LS and/or MMR gene variant carriers are diagnosed accurately and receive appropriate surveillance as individuals with a high risk of cancer. However, it is expected that a greater number of these cases will be picked up through comprehensive genome screening represented by cancer gene panels.

Thus, the importance of understanding this syndrome will increase rapidly in the future.

On the publication of this special edition of *Lynch Syndrome: Molecular Mechanisms and Current Topics*, I aimed to clearly present our latest understanding of this important clinical entity, "Lynch syndrome," and thus selected 13 chapters and invited 13 experts in this field from Japan. Among these 13 authors, gastrointestinal surgeons, basic researchers, and a gastroenterologist, gastrointestinal endoscopist, gynecologist, urologist, pathologist, cancer geneticist, and epidemiologist are contained. The fact that this feature includes authors encompassing various fields is exactly a reflection of the nature of hereditary cancer syndromes, especially that of LS.

This book presents the most recent findings of the molecular mechanisms and current topics of the diagnosis and treatment for this disease.

I hope this cutting-edge review of LS will provide readers with the latest information in one concise source.

Lastly, I would like to add one more important message.

It is widely known that Prof. Henry T. Lynch passed away on June 2, 2019, at the age of 91 years. He was not only a pioneer of cancer genetics as an excellent researcher but was also a dedicated clinician for patients and great teacher for us all. Dr. Lynch visited Japan several times, imparting a significant influence on and great contribution to the field of hereditary cancers in Japan.

I would like to dedicate this book to the late Prof. Henry T. Lynch.

References

1. Warthin AS. Heredity with reference to carcinoma as shown by the study of the cases examined in the pathological laboratory of the University of Michigan, 1895–1913. Arch Intern Med. 1913;12:546–55.
2. Lynch HT, Shaw MW, Magnuson CW, et al. Hereditary factors in cancer. Study of two large Midwestern kindreds. Arch Intern Med. 1966;117:206–12.
3. Lynch HT, Lanspa S, Shaw T, et al. Phenotypic and genotypic heterogeneity of Lynch syndrome: a complex diagnostic challenge. Familial Cancer 2017 Oct 25. 2017. https://doi.org/10.1007/s10689-017-0053-3. [Epub ahead of print].
4. Japanese Society for the Colon and Rectum (JSCCR) Guidelines 2016 for the Clinical Practice of Hereditary Colorectal Cancer. 1st ed. Tokyo (in Japanese).
5. Ishida H, Yamaguchi T, Tanakaya K, et al. Japanese Society for Cancer of the Colon and Rectum (JSCCR) Guidelines 2016 for the Clinical Practice of Hereditary Colorectal Cancer (Translated Version). J Anus Rectum Colon. 2018;2(Suppl. I):S1–51.

Toyonaka, Osaka, Japan
Nishinomiya, Hyogo, Japan

Naohiro Tomita

Contents

Molecular Mechanism of Lynch Syndrome

1

Kazuo Tamura

Abstract

Lynch syndrome is a cancer-predisposing syndrome inherited in an autosomal dominant manner, wherein colon cancer and endometrial cancer develop frequently in the family, it results from a loss of function of one of four different protein (MLH1, MSH2, MSH6, and PMS2), which are the products of mismatch repair genes. An abnormal *EPCAM* gene at the position adjacent to the *MSH2* gene also inhibits *MSH2* expression and causes Lynch syndrome.

Mismatch repair proteins are involved in repairing of incorrect pairing, including point mutations and deletion/insertion of simple repetitive sequences, so-called microsatellites, that can arise during DNA replication. MSH2 forms heterodimers with MSH6 or MSH3 (MutSα, MutSβ, respectively) and is involved in mismatch-pair recognition and initiation of repair. MLH1 forms a complex with PMS2 and functions as an endonuclease. If the mismatch repair system is thoroughly working, genome integrity is maintained at a high level. Lynch syndrome is a state of mismatch repair deficiency (MMRd) due to a monoallelic abnormality of the mismatch repair genes. The phenotype indicating the mismatch repair deficiency can be frequently observed as a microsatellite instability (MSI) in tumors.

Generally, Lynch syndrome develops in adulthood, but MMR gene abnormalities are observed in children with different genotypes and phenotypes. Children with germline biallelic mismatch repair gene abnormalities were reported to develop conditions such as gastrointestinal polyposis, colorectal cancer, brain cancer, leukemia, and so on. This condition is called constitutional mismatch repair deficiency (CMMRD).

K. Tamura (✉)
Division of Medical Genetics, Master of Science, Graduate School of Science and Engineering Research, Kindai University, Higashiosaka, Japan

Genetic and Genomic Medical Center, Sakurabashi- Watanabe Hospital, Osaka, Japan
e-mail: tamura@life.kindai.ac.jp

N. Tomita (ed.), *Lynch Syndrome*, https://doi.org/10.1007/978-981-15-6891-6_1

In addition, for promoting cancer genome medicine in a new era, such as by utilizing immune checkpoints, it is important to understand the genetic and genomic molecular background, including the status of mismatch repair deficiency.

Keywords

Mismatch repair gene · Lynch syndrome · Microsatellite instability · Constitutional mismatch repair deficiency · Immune checkpoint inhibitor

Abbreviation

CMMR-D	Constitutional mismatch repair deficiency
CNS	Central nervous system
CTE	Congenital tufting enteropathy
CTLA-4	Cytotoxic T-lymphocyte-associated protein 4
IHC	Immunohistochemical staining
ISI	Immune checkpoint inhibitor
MLPA	Multiple ligation-dependent probe amplification
MMR	Mismatch repair
MSI	Microsatellite instability
PCNA	Proliferating cellular nuclear antigen
PD-1	Programmed cell death protein 1
RFC	Replication factor
TMB	Tumor mutational burden

1.1 Introduction

Cancer is fundamentally a genetic disease, and pathogenic variants, also called "mutation," are pivotal to its etiology and progression. Carcinogenesis develops by the accumulation of numerous genetic and epigenetic abnormalities [1–4]. Therefore, cancer has the following six characteristics: sustained proliferative signaling, evasion of growth suppressors, resistance cell death, replicative immortality, angiogenesis induction, and activation of invasion and metastasis [5]. Therefore, elucidation of carcinogenesis is essential for therapeutic development [6]. Although rare, hereditary cancer syndromes are observed in cancers derived from any organ. In individuals with hereditary cancer syndrome, the initial cancer-causing pathogenic variant is inherited through the germ cell and therefore, is already present in all 37 trillion cells that make up the body. Lynch syndrome (MIM# 120435) is an autosomal dominant syndrome with a penetration rate of about 80% characterized by several individuals in the family affected with colorectal cancer (CRC) or extracolonic tumors of the endometrium, stomach, small bowel, ureter, renal pelvis, ovary, and hepatobiliary tract [7].

Lynch syndrome occurs due to loss of function of the mismatch repair mechanism for genomic replication errors. This article outlines the basis of molecular genetics involved in Lynch syndrome.

1.2 DNA Repair System

The frequency of replication errors is 10^{-10} per base of DNA per cell division, and in an estimated 10^{15} cell divisions during an individual's lifetime replication errors cause thousands of new DNA variants in the genome in every cell. Eukaryotes have multiple repair systems to avoid replication errors (Table 1.1) [8]. Maintaining DNA-integrity through genome repair suppresses cancer development and progression by genomic abnormalities. Genes encoding molecules involved in genome repair are referred to as DNA repair genes and "caretaker tumor suppressor genes."

Table 1.1 DNA repair systems and predisposition to cancer [8]

DNA repair	Damage	Characteristics	Predisposition
Base excision Repair (BER)	Single strand	Repair mechanism for a single nucleotide in a single strand of DNA that is generated through oxidation (e.g., 8-oxoguanine), alkylation (e.g., methylation), and deamination. No ATP required	*MUTYH*-associated polyposis (MAP)
Nucleotide excision repair (NER)	Single strand	Repair mechanism against damage that causes DNA structure change over several tens of base pairs via pyrimidine dimer formation by ultraviolet exposure. ATP required	Xeroderma pigmentosum Cockayne Syndrome
Mismatch repair: (MMR)	Single strand	Repair mechanism of base mismatch pairing caused in DNA replication (S phase). Usually, it corresponds to an error of one to several base pairs ATP required	Lynch syndrome
Proofreading repair	Single strand	It occurs done during DNA replication. In E. coli, 3′→5′ exonuclease of DNA polymerase I has this function. In humans, involvement of enzymes other than DNA polymerase is also conceivable	Polymerase proofreading associated polyposis (PPAP)
Homologous recombination (HR)	Double strand	When double stranded breaks occur in S phase/G2 phase, the cleaved portion of a normal allele is used as the template DNA. This mechanism restores the original sequence by recombination	Hereditary breast and ovarian cancer (HBOC)
Nonhomologous end-Joining (NHEJ)	Double strand	In double strand breaks in the G1 phase, this repair mechanism concentrates multiple molecules on the excised ends and directly combines them. In this repair, some nucleotides around the break part may be missing in some cases	LIG4 syndrome

Table 1.2 DNA repair system for replication errors in *Esherichia coli* [8]

Step	Pathway	Protein activities	Mutation rate (per nucleotide per generation)
1	DNA synthesis	5′→3′-elongation activity of DNA polymerase III(α) (1000 nucleotides/s.)	10^{-5}–10^{-6}
2	Proofreading	3′→5′-exonuclease activity of DNA polymerase III(ε)	10^{-7}
3	Mismatch correction	Mismatch correction proteins Mut S, Mut L, Mut H etc.	10^{-9}–10^{-10}

The mismatch repair system was recognized in 1961, with proposal that the correction of DNA base pair mismatches within recombination intermediates is the basis for gene conversion [9]. Elucidation of the mismatch repair system has been advanced by fundamental research based on *Escherichia coli*, developed four *E. coli* mutator genes: *mutH*, *mutL*, *mutS*, and *uvrD* [10–13]. Inactivation of any of these genes increases the generation of variants in the *E. coli* cell by 50-to 100-fold, indicating the importance of this pathway in variant avoidance and genetic stability. The reduction in mutability afforded by the *E. coli* methyl-directed system has been attributed to its role in the strand-specific elimination of DNA errors (Table 1.2) [6, 8, 14–19]. Research on the mismatch repair system has advanced extensively and has clarified its mechanism and role as an essential mechanism for maintaining genome integrity in organisms and involved in predisposition to cancer development.

1.3 Genes Responsible for Lynch Syndrome

Lynch syndrome, is called hereditary nonpolyposis colorectal cancer: HNPCC in the past, is an autosomal dominant inherited disorder caused by germline pathogenic variants in DNA mismatch repair (MMR) genes. Patients with Lynch syndrome are at an increased risk of developing tumors from a young age and throughout their lifetime. Most of them suffer from multiple synchronous and/or metachronous primary tumors. Colorectal cancer and endometrial cancer (female) are well known in the tumor spectrum of Lynch syndrome. In addition, patients with Lynch syndrome have high potential for developing cancer of the urinary tract, the stomach, the small intestine, the biliary tract, the skin, the brain, and others.

Multiple types of human mismatch repair (MMR) proteins have been discovered and several encoding genes have been isolated so far. Currently, four types of MMR genes, *MLH1* (MIM# 120436), *MSH2* (MIM# 609309), *MSH6* (MIM# 600678), and *PMS2* (MIM# 600259), are used in the clinical applications related to Lynch syndrome. An outline of the responsible genes is shown in Fig. 1.1. The *EPCAM*, which encodes a cell adhesion molecule, is not an MMR gene, but its structural abnormality causes Lynch syndrome, because it is adjacent to the *MSH2* gene [20]. This content will be described later.

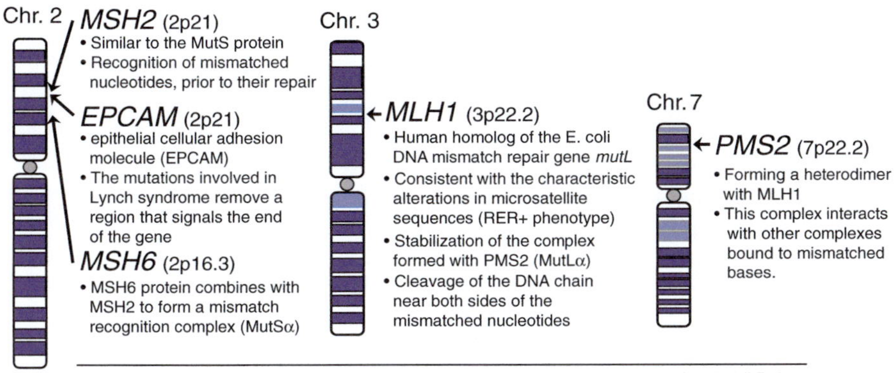

Gene	MIM	Locus	No.of exon	CDS (nt)	Product no. of amino acid	MW (kDa) of protein
MLH1	*120436	3p22.2	19	2218	756	84.6
MSH2	*609309	2p21	16	2802	934	104.7
MSH6	*600678	2p16.3	10	4080	1360	152.8
PMS2	*600259	7p22.1	15	2586	862	95.8
EPCAM	*185535	2p21	9	942	314	35

Fig. 1.1 The genes responsible for Lynch syndrome [8]

In 1993, *MSH2* gene was isolated at chromosome 2p22–p21 in 1993 and has high homology with the mutator phenotype gene, mutS of *E. coli* [21–24]. In 1994, as the second responsible gene of Lynch syndrome, *MLH1*, the *E. coli mutL* homologue, was isolated from 3p22.2 [25–27]. In 1995, mismatch binding factors were found as the 100 kD MSH2 or as heterodimers of the 160 kD polypeptide called GTBP/MSH6 (for G/T binding protein), which was recognized as a new member of the MutS homologue [28, 29]. *MSH6* gene was first reported by Japanese researchers as a gene responsible for Lynch syndrome [30, 31]. In 1994, a germline deletion of the *PMS2* was also identified in families with Lynch syndrome. Moreover, additional deletions in tumor samples with microsatellite instability high (MSI-high) showed the presence of two-hits [32, 33].

1.4 Structure and Function of MMR Proteins

Each MMR protein encoded by the corresponding MMR gene has a unique function in repairing replication errors. Therefore, MMR proteins possess unique functional domains. When pathogenic variants of MMR genes occur in the DNA site corresponding to the functional domain, DNA repair function may be impaired. Schematic representations of MLH1, MSH2, MSH6, and PMS2 proteins are shown in Fig. 1.2 [8, 34–38]. Both MLH1 and PMS2 have an ATP binding domain and require ATP molecules for the endonuclease function.

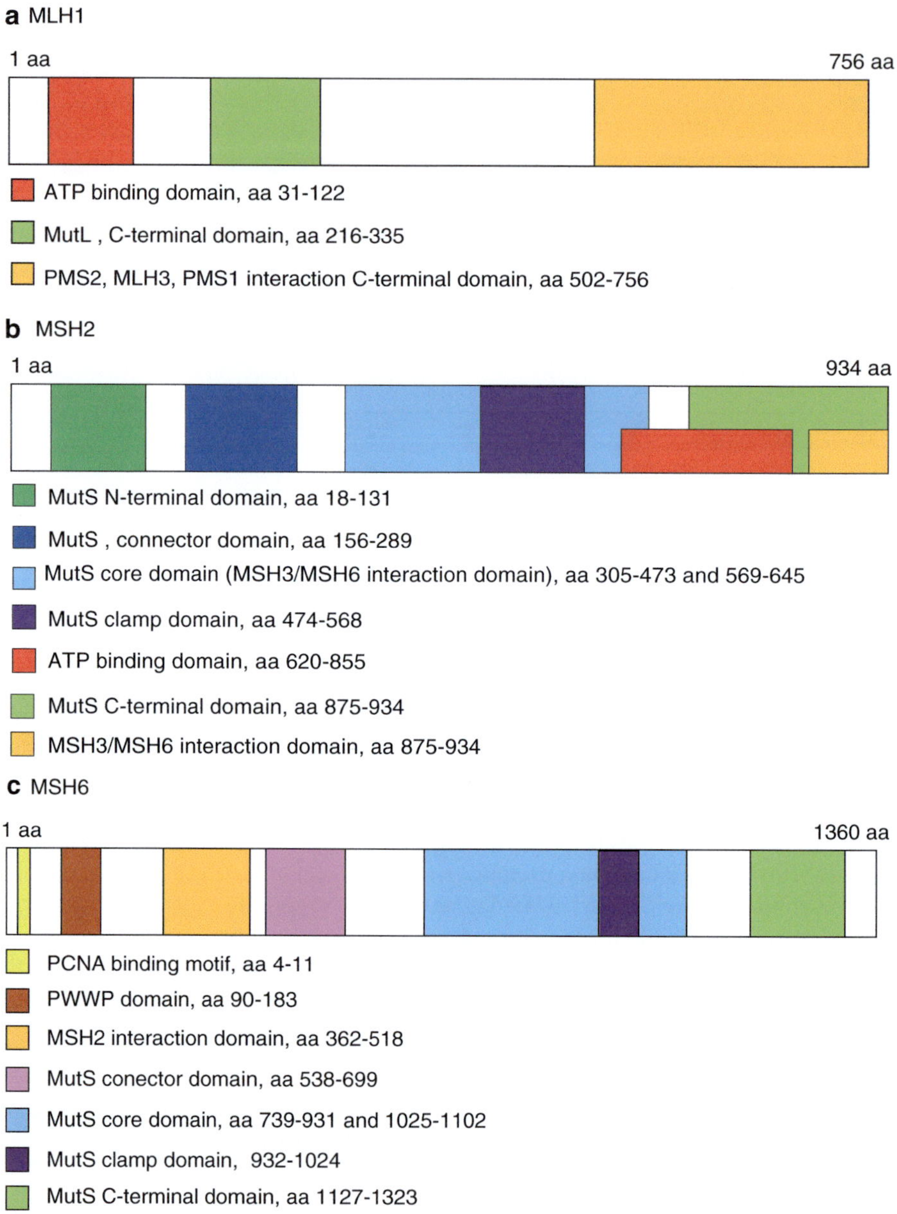

Fig. 1.2 Structure of mismatch repair proteins (**a**) *MLH1*, (**b**) *MSH2*, (**c**) *MSH6*, (**d**) *PMS2* [8]

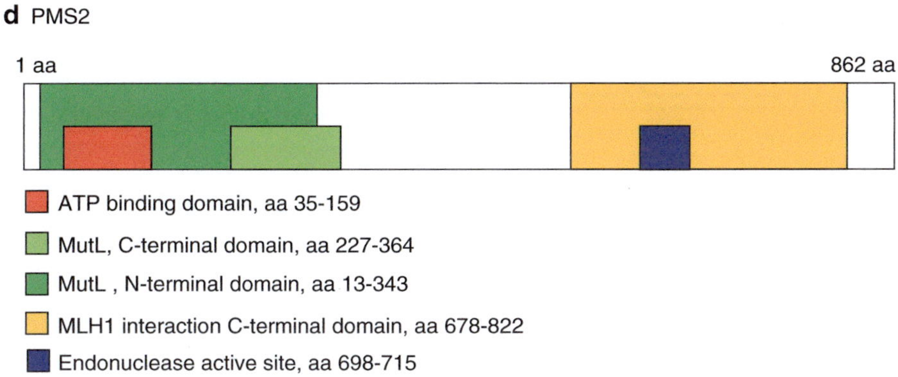

Fig. 1.2 (continued)

Many human MMR related proteins have been identified as homologues of *E. coli* MMR proteins [8, 22–29, 39–49]. These include human homologues of MutS, MutL, ExoI, DNA polymerase δ (pol δ), proliferating cellular nuclear antigen (PCNA), replication factor (RFC), DNA ligase I, and so on. MSH2 heterodimerizes with MSH6 or MSH3 to form MutSα or MutSβ, respectively. These are involved in the mismatch-pair recognition and initiation of repair [50–54]. In addition, various kinds of complexes such as MutLα, MutLβ, and MutLγ are formed and involved in the mismatch repair system [37, 38, 40, 51, 52, 54–63].

1.5 Mechanisms of Mismatch Repair

The mismatch repair (MMR) system consists of sequential steps for the recognition, removal, and resynthesis of the mismatch site in DNA. This system that maintains DNA fidelity is well conserved from *E. coli* to eukaryotes. A schematic diagram of the pathway is shown in Fig. 1.3 [8, 53, 58, 60, 62–82]. Base–base mismatches in double-strand DNA are recognized by MutSα (heterodimer of MSH2-MSH6). MutSα binds as a sliding clamp around the double-strand DNA. MutSα and MutLα form a tetrameric complex and then initiate the process of mismatch repair. The tetrameric complex recruits proliferating cell nuclear antigen (PCNA), replication factor C (RFC), exonuclease 1 (Exo 1) to remove the nascent (daughter) strand, and resynthesize the correct strand. Then, exonuclease 1 (Exo 1) is recruited and removes the nascent (daughter) strand around the error region. The resynthesis step is accomplished by DNA polymerase (Polδ or Polε) and Ligase 1.

1.6 Relationship Between MMR System and DNA Damages

Depending on the DNA damage pattern, specific mismatch repair molecules, and complexes are involved. The outline is shown in Fig. 1.4 [8, 50, 64, 66, 83–86]. The MutSα (heterodimer of MSH2-MSH6) contributes to mismatch recognition by

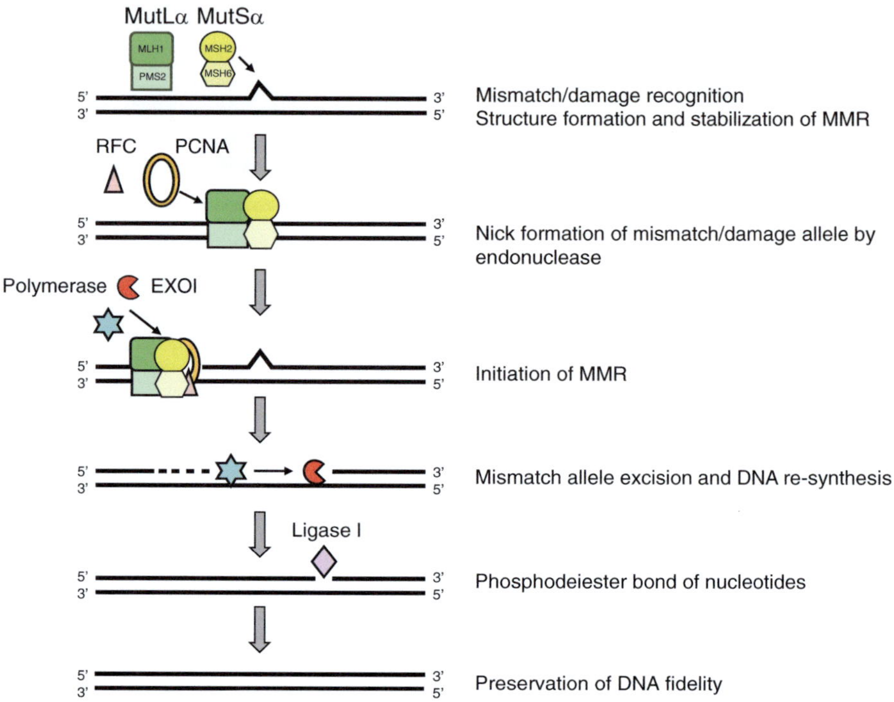

Fig. 1.3 Mechanistic model of mismatch repair [8]

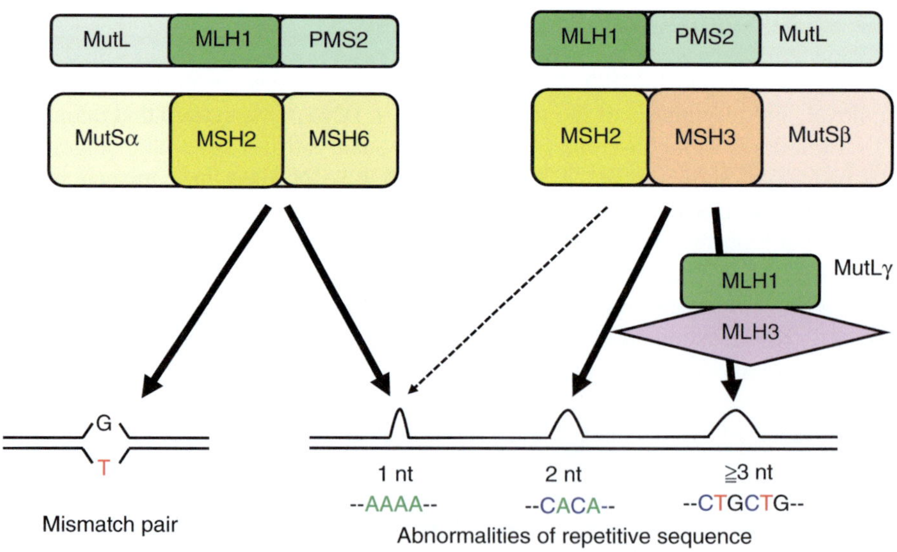

Fig. 1.4 Schematic of DNA damage recognized by the mismatch repair pathway [8]

single nucleotide substitution (e.g., G:T mismatch pair) and recognition of small insertion-deletion loops (IDL, e.g., error of the repeat number in adenine clusters), whereas MutSβ (heterodimer of MSH2-MSH3) contributes to the repair of small loops and relatively large damages up to about ten nucleotide loops. Recently, the function of MutSβ has attracted attention for its biological characteristics and as a prognostic factor of elevated microsatellite instability at selected tetranucleotide (EMAST) colorectal cancer, which shows instability in the repeat sequence of the tetranucleotides [87–91].

1.7 *EPCAM* as the Gene Responsible for Lynch Syndrome

EPCAM is located at 2p21 adjacent to the *MSH2* on the 5′ upstream and encodes the EPCAM protein, expressed on the membrane of cells in epithelial tissues and plasma cells, and is involved in cell-cell adhesion function [92, 93]. Although *EPCAM* is not the direct responsible gene of Lynch syndrome, but it is located just 17 kb upstream of *MSH2*. The deletion of *EPCAM* affects *MSH2* gene expression, resulting in Lynch syndrome. The schema is shown in Fig. 1.5 [8, 20]. The *cis*-deleted alleles inhibit *MSH2* expression and finally causes Lynch syndrome in 1.3% of the affected families [20, 94].

In addition, biallelic inactivation of *EPCAM* is responsible for congenital tufting enteropathy (CTE, MIM# 613217) with an estimated incidence of one in 50,000–100,000 births in Western Europe [95–98]. CTE presents within the first months of life with severe chronic watery diarrhea and growth restriction. *EPCAM* abnormalities responsible for CTE are usually missense mutations, nonsense mutations, minute insertions/deletions, and splicing errors, unlike Lynch syndrome [98].

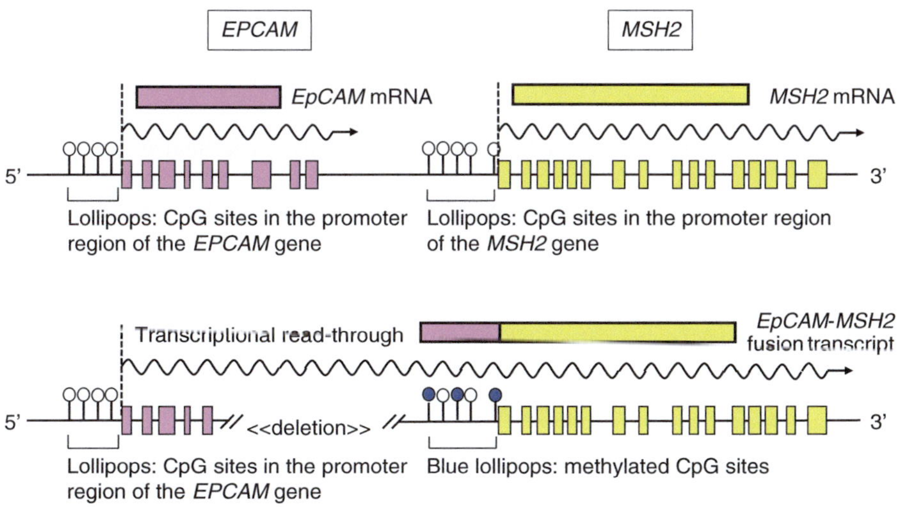

Fig. 1.5 A *cis*-deletion of *EPCAM* gene causes an epimutation of the *MSH2* gene [8]

1.8 Constitutional Mismatch Repair Deficiency Syndrome

Constitutional mismatch repair deficiency syndrome (CMMR-D) is caused by biallelic homozygous or compound heterozygous pathogenic germline pathogenic variants of MMR genes and is a distinct childhood cancer preposition syndrome (MIM# 276300) with an autosomal recessive inheritance [99–101]. In biallelic germline pathogenic variant carriers of MMR genes, hematological malignancies, brain/central nervous system (CNS) tumors, and Lynch syndrome associated carcinomas develop frequently. In the gastrointestinal tract, bowel adenomatous polyposes are often observed as premalignant lesions that require differential diagnosis from FAP. By the way, the pathological condition classified as a subtype of FAP called Turcot's syndrome is considered to be exactly CMRR-D [102, 103].

The median age at diagnosis of hematological malignancies and brain/CNS tumors was respectively, 6.6 (age range: 1.2–30.8) and 10.3 (age range: 3.3–40) years. However, Lynch syndrome-associated tumors developed later (median age at diagnosis: 21.4 years (age range: 11.4–36.6)). Moreover, the spectrum of Lynch syndrome is mostly colorectal cancer and/or endometrial cancer [104]. Various non-neoplastic features are related to CMMR-D including Cafe au lait spots (NF1 like), skin hypopigmentation, mild defects in immunoglobulin class switching recombination, agenesis of the corpus callosum, cavernous brain hemangioma, capillary hemangioma of the skin, combination of various congenital malformations, and lupus erythematosus.

1.9 Genetic Testing for Lynch Syndrome

In order to select high-risk individuals with Lynch syndrome from among patients with colorectal cancer and to increase the efficiency of detecting germline pathogenic variants, microsatellite instability (MSI) testing and/or immunohistochemical staining (IHC) of MMR proteins is recommended as universal tumor screening and is recommended to do first [102, 105, 106]. The MSI testing is a method to easily identify events in which genetic integrity has been damaged due to repair failures of DNA replication errors using simple repeated microsatellite sequences [107–111]. Five types of repeat markers including mononucleotide and dinucleotide repeats have been used, but recently mononucleotide repeat markers have been preferred. Cases with different numbers of repeats between normal tissue-derived DNA and cancer-derived DNA are considered as positive [112]. If two or more of the five markers show instability, the tumor is evaluated as MSI-high (MSI-H). The results of MSI-H colorectal cancer are shown in Fig. 1.6. If one of the markers shows instability, the tumor is considered as MSI-low (MSI-L). If positive markers are not observed, the mismatch repair system is evaluated to be proficient and is called MS-stable (MSS).

Immunohistochemical staining of MMR proteins can reveal damaged molecules using specific antibodies. Staining with four antibodies: MLH1, MSH2, MSH6, and PMS2 can predict the gene causing Lynch syndrome (Table 1.3) [113–120].

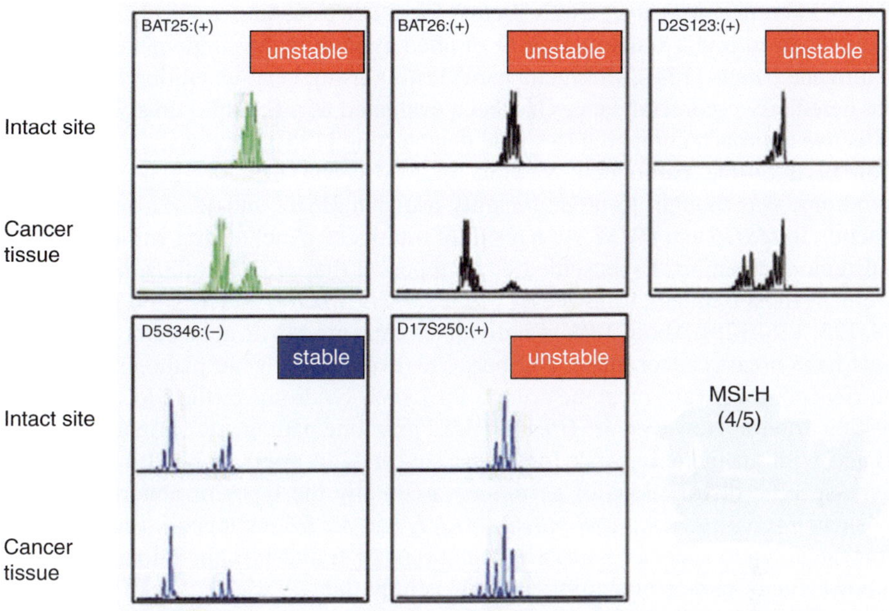

Fig. 1.6 Analytic image of MSI testing: four out of five markers show microsatellite instability [8]

Table 1.3 IHC findings associated with *MLH1*, *MSH2*, *MSH6*, and *PMS2* mutations [8]

	IHC staining			
Mutation of MMR genes	MLH1	MSH2	MSH6	PMS2
MLH1	–	+	+	–
MSH2	+	–	–	+
MSH6	+	+	–	+
PMS2	+	+	+	–

For MSI testing, sensitivity ranged from 66.7 to 100.0% and specificity ranged from 61.1 to 92.5%, whereas for IHC staining, sensitivity ranged from 80.8 to 100.0%, and specificity ranged from 80.5 to 91.9% [121].

Approximately 10–15% of sporadic colorectal cancers show MSI-H findings. The cause is mostly the loss of MSH1 protein due to methylation of the *MLH1* gene promoter region. About half of MSI-H sporadic colorectal cancers show *BRAF* V600E mutation, which is rarely detected in colorectal cancers from patients with Lynch syndrome. *MLH1* methylation analysis and *BRAF* V600E mutation testing in colorectal cancers can improve the efficiency of the diagnosis for Lynch syndrome [36, 122].

Final genetic testing for Lynch syndrome is performed using DNA sequencing in selected cases excluding sporadic colon cancer from all colorectal cancers. For a long time, genetic testing has mainly been performed using Sanger sequencing, and multiplex ligation-dependent probe amplification (MLPA) has been adopted for a wide range of abnormalities such as large deletions/insertions [123]. Clinical genetics is currently transitioning from phenotype-directed single gene testing to multigene panels [124]. Multigene panel testing using next generation sequencing for hereditary colorectal cancer has been evaluated as a feasible, timely, and cost-effective approach compared to single gene testing [125]. Previously, the distribution of germline pathogenic variants in MMR and *EPCAM* genes in Lynch syndrome was thought to predominantly occur in *MSH2* and *MLH1* and less frequently in *MSH6* and *PMS2*. As a result of multigene panel testing without universal tumor screening, Espenschied et al. reported that *MSH6* pathogenic variants were the most frequent, followed by *PMS2*, *MSH2*, *MLH1*, and *EPCAM* (Table 1.4) [8, 123, 126–128]. About 12% of individuals carrying MMR gene pathogenic variants have breast cancer alone. Furthermore, even MMR gene pathogenic variant carriers do not always meet the criteria for Lynch syndrome or the *BRCA1*/*BRCA2* testing criteria. However, *MSH6* and *PMS2* germline pathogenic variants are associated with an increased risk for breast cancer [126, 129]. Table 1.4 shows the gene-specific distributions of germline variants by the types of abnormalities in mismatch repair genes. Most *MSH2*, *MLH1*, and *MSH6* pathogenic variants were truncated types such as nonsense mutations or frameshift mutations [8, 130]. Knowledge of choice of analysis method is important. A wide range of rearrangements were detected at 10%, 7%, and 10% for MSH2, MLH1, and PMS2, respectively. Therefore, the selection of an appropriate analysis method is required for genetic testing.

Table 1.4 Germline mutation analyses in the responsible genes in Lynch syndrome [8]

(a) Distribution of mutations in overall mismatch repair genes and *EPCAM*

Gene	*MSH2* (%)	*MLH1* (%)	*MSH6* (%)	*PMS2* (%)	*EPCAM* (%)	Publication year	Ref#
Distribution of mutations in overall mismatch repair genes and *EPCAM* gene	23.7	21.6	29.4	24.2	1.2	2017	[126]
	21.2	39.4	18.2	21.2	–	2017	[127]
	36	40	18	6	–	2016	[128]
	34	40	18	8	–	2014	[129]

(b) Distribution of the types of germline variants in mismatch repair genes [130]

Variant type	*MSH2* (%)	*MLH1* (%)	*MSH6* (%)	*PMS2* (%)
Missense	31	40	49	62
Nonsense or frameshift	49	40	43	24
In-frame	2	2	3	1
Splice	8	11	3	3
Large rearrangement	10	7	2	10

1.10 Effectiveness of Immune Check Point Blockades and a Hypermutable State (High Tumor Mutational Burden)

As cancer cells escape the host immune system by suppressing T cell activation, thus exert an immunosuppressive function due to immune checkpoint molecules. The immune checkpoint molecules include cytotoxic T-lymphocyte-associated protein 4 (CTLA-4) and programmed cell death protein 1 (PD-1, CD279), and so on [131, 132], which were found to negatively control the immune system [133, 134]. In human cancer treatment, anti-PD-1 antibody was found to be effective for non-small cell lung cancer, malignant melanoma, and renal cell cancer and was also clinically applicable in safety [135]. The clinical efficacy of PD-1 inhibitor was found to be higher in mismatch repair-defective colorectal and non-colorectal cancers compared to proficient-mismatch repair cancers [136]. According to recent survey results, as shown in Fig. 1.7, high tumor mutational burden (TMB) is an excellent biomarker for predicting the efficacy of immune checkpoint inhibitors (ICIs) [137–139], and the group of colorectal cancer patients with the biological characteristics of mismatch repair deficient (MMRd) has a significantly better response to ICIs

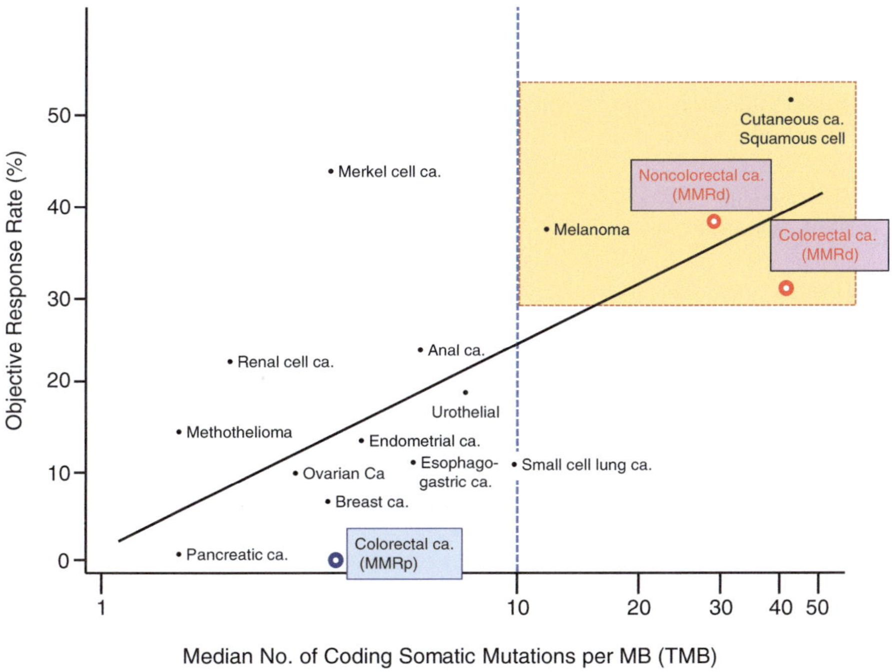

Fig. 1.7 Correlation between tumor mutational burden (TMB) and objective response rate with immune checkpoint inhibitors [137]

than those with mismatch repair proficient (MMRp) [136, 137]. In gastrointestinal cancer, because the state of microsatellite instability high (MSI-H) state has been shown to correlate well with high TMB based on an analysis of many cancer genomes, the microsatellite instability (MSI) testing is used as a standard biomarker to predict the response of ICIs [140–142].

1.11 Future Directions

The cancer-accumulating family reported by Warthin AS more than 100 years ago led to the establishment of Lynch syndrome by the vigorous genetic epidemiological approach of Lynch HT et al. On the other hand, mismatch repair genes have been elucidated as part of the genome integrity system of *Escherichia col*i and yeast. These basic researchers worked together to understand the clinical, genetic, and molecular biological aspects of Lynch syndrome. With its natural history and molecular biological characteristics clarified, presymptomatic diagnosis by genetic testing for at-risk persons in the family, and appropriate medically actionable interventions, such as early diagnosis, are becoming possible.

The development of ICIs is a major milestone in the treatment of patients with Lynch Syndrome. Most malignant tumors in patients with LS have MSI-H status and are expected to respond to ICIs. These studies have shown new possibilities for the treatment of hereditary tumor syndrome. In future, we hope that advances in the integrated understanding of the clinical and molecular biology of Lynch syndrome will lead to the development of novel diagnostic methods and effective treatments.

Acknowledgments This work was supported in part by a grant from the Japanese Ministry of Education, Science, Sports and Culture of Japan (19K07763).

Disclosure Statement of COI

The author declares no potential conflicts of interest.

ORCID: https://orcid.org/0000-0002-1087-9851

References

1. Vogelstein B, Fearon ER, Hamilton SR, et al. Genetic alterations during colorectal-tumor development. N Engl J Med. 1988;319:525–32.
2. Fearon ER, Vogelstein B. A genetic model for colorectal tumorigenesis. Cell. 1990;61:759–67.
3. Bodmer W, Bishop T, Karran P. Genetic steps in colorectal cancer. Nat Genet. 1994;6:217–9.
4. Kinzler KW, Vogelstein B. Lessons from hereditary colorectal cancer. Cell. 1996;87:159–70.
5. Hanahan D, Weinberg RA. Hallmarks of cancer: the next generation. Cell. 2011;144:646–74.
6. Tamura K, Utsunomiya J, Iwama T, et al. Mechanism of carcinogenesis in familial tumors. Int J Clin Oncol. 2004;9:232–45.
7. Lynch HT, de la Chapelle A. Hereditary colorectal cancer. N Engl J Med. 2003;348:919–32.
8. Tamura K, Kaneda M, Futagawa M, et al. Genetic and genomic basis of the mismatch repair system involved in Lynch syndrome. Int J Clin Oncol. 2019;24:999–1011.

9. Holliday R. A mechanism for gene conversion in fungi. Genet Res. 1964;5:282–304.
10. Modrich P. Mechanisms in *E. coli* and mismatch repair. Angew Chem Int Ed Engl. 2016;55:8490–501.
11. Nevers P, Spats HC. *Escherichia coli* mutants uvr D and uvr E deficient in gene conversion of lambda-heteroduplexes. Mol Gen Genet. 1975;139:233–43.
12. Rydberg B. Bromouracil mutagenesis and mismatch repair in mutator strains of *Esherichia coli*. Mutat Res. 1978;52:11–24.
13. Glickman BW, Radman M. *Esherichia coli* mutator mutants deficient in methylation-instructed DNA mismatch correction. Proc Natl Acad Sci U S A. 1980;77:1063–7.
14. Lauhe RS, Su SS, Morich P. Requirement for d(GATC) sequences in *Esherichia coli mutHLS* mismatch correction. Proc Natl Acad Sci U S A. 1987;84:1482–6.
15. Su SS, Morrich P. *Esherichia coli mutS*-encoded protein binds to mismatched DNA base pairs. Proc Natl Acad Sci USA. 1986;83:5057–61.
16. Meselson M. Methyl-directed repair of DNA mismatches. In: Low KB, editor. Recombination of the genetic material. San Diego, CA: Academic Press; 1988. p. 91–113.
17. Modrich P. Methyl-directed DNA mismatch correction. J Biol Chem. 1989;264:6597–600.
18. Grilley M, Holmes J, Yashar B, et al. Mechanisms of DNA-mismatch correction. Mutat Res. 1990;236:253–67.
19. Modrich P. Mechanisms and biological effects of mismatch repair. Annu Rev Genet. 1991;25:229–53.
20. Ligtenberg MJL, Kuiper RP, Chan TL, et al. Heritable somatic methylation and inactivation of *MSH2* in families with Lynch syndrome due to deletion of the 3-prime exons of *TACSTD1*. Nat Genet. 2009;41:112–7.
21. Fishel R, Lescoe MK, Rao MRS, et al. The human mutator gene homolog *MSH2* and its association. Cell. 1993;75:1027–38.
22. Leach FS, Nicolaides NC, Papadopoulos N, et al. Mutations of a *mutS* homolog in hereditary nonpolyposis colorectal cancer. Cell. 1993;75:1215–25.
23. Kolodner RD, Hall NR, Lipford J, et al. Structure of the human *MSH2* locus and analysis of two Muir-Torre kindreds for *msh2* mutations. Genomics. 1994;24:516–26.
24. Fishel R, Ewel A, Lee S, et al. Binding of mismatched microsatellite DNA sequences by the human MSH2 protein. Science. 1993;266:1403–5.
25. Papadopoulos N, Nicolaides NC, Wei Y-F, et al. Mutation of a mutL homolog in hereditary colon cancer. Science. 1994;263:1625–9.
26. Bronner CE, Baker SM, Morrison PT, et al. Mutation in the DNA mismatch repair gene homologue *hMLH1* is associated with hereditary non-polyposis colon cancer. Nature. 1994;368:258–61.
27. Han H-J, Maruyama M, Baba S, et al. Genomic structure of human mismatch repair gene, *hMLH1*, and its mutation analysis in patients with hereditary non-polyposis colorectal cancer (HNPCC). Hum Mol Genet. 1995;4:237–42.
28. Drummond JT, Li G-M, Longley MJ, et al. Isolation of an hMSH2-p160 heterodimer that restores DNA mismatch repair to tumor cells. Science. 1995;268:1909–12.
29. Palombo F, Gallinari P, Iaccarino I, et al. GTBP, a 160-kilodalton protein essential for mismatch-binding activity in human cells. Science. 1995;268:1912–4.
30. Miyaki M, Konishi M, Tanaka K, et al. Germline mutation of *MSH6* as the cause of hereditary nonpolyposis colorectal cancer. Nat Genet. 1997;17:271–2.
31. Akiyama Y, Sato H, Yamada T, et al. Germ-line mutation of the hMSH6/GTBP gene in an atypical hereditary nonpolyposis colorectal cancer kindred. Cancer Res. 1997;57:3920–3.
32. Nicolaides NC, Papadopoulos N, Liu B, et al. Mutations of two *PMS* homologues in hereditary nonpolyposis colon cancer. Nature. 1994;371:75–80.
33. De Vos M, Hayward BE, Picton S, et al. Novel *PMS2* pseudogenes can conceal recessive mutations causing a distinctive childhood cancer syndrome. Am J Hum Genet. 2004;74:954–64.
34. Ban C, Juno M, Yang W. Transformation of MutL by ATP binding and hydrolysis: a switch in DNA mismatch repair. Cell. 1999;97:85–97.

35. Tran PT, Liskay RM. Functional studies on the candidate ATPase domains of *Saccharomyces cerevisiae* MutLalpha. Mol Cell Biol. 2000;20:6390–8.
36. Räschle M, Dufner P, Marra G, et al. Mutations within the *hMLH1* and *hPMS2* subunits of the human MutLalpha mismatch repair factor affect its ATPase activity, but not its ability to interact with hMutSalpha. J Biol Chem. 2002;277:21810–20.
37. Guerrette S, Acharya S, Fishel R. The interaction of the human MutL homologues in hereditary nonpolyposis colon cancer. J Biol Chem. 1999;274:6336–41.
38. Kondo E, Horii A, Fukushige S. The interaction domains of three MutL heterodimers in man: hMLH1 interacts with 36 homologous amino acid residues within hMLH3, hPMS1 and hPMS2. Nucleic Acids Res. 2001;29:1695–708.
39. Reenan RA, Kolodner RD. Isolation and characterization of two Saccharomyces cerevisiae genes encoding homologs of the bacterial HexA and MutS mismatch repair proteins. Genetics. 1992;132:963–73.
40. Li GM, Modrich P. Restoration of mismatch repair to nuclear extracts of H6 colorectal tumor cells by a heterodimer of human MutL homologs. Proc Natl Acad Sci U S A. 1995;92:1950–4.
41. Johnson RE, Kovvali GK, Guzder SN, et al. Evidence for involvement of yeast proliferating cell nuclear antigen in DNA mismatch repair. J Biol Chem. 1996;271:27987–90.
42. Umar A, Buermeyer AB, Simon JA, et al. Requirement for PCNA in DNA mismatch repair at a step preceding DNA resynthesis. Cell. 1996;87:65–73.
43. Tishkoff DX, Boerger AL, Bertrand P, et al. Identification and characterization of Saccharomyces cerevisiae EXO1, a gene encoding an exonuclease that interacts with MSH2. Proc Natl Acad Sci U S A. 1997;94:7487–92.
44. Longley MJ, Pierce AJ, Modrich P. DNA polymerase delta is required for human mismatch repair in vitro. J Biol Chem. 1997;272:10917–21.
45. Schmutte C, Marinescu RC, Sadoff MM, et al. Human exonuclease I interacts with the mismatch repair protein hMSH2. Cancer Res. 1998;58:4537–42.
46. Tishkoff DX, Amin NS, Viars CS, et al. Identification of a human gene encoding a homologue of *Saccharomyces cerevisiae* EXO1, an exonuclease implicated in mismatch repair and recombination. Cancer Res. 1998;58:5027–31.
47. Lin YL, Shivji MK, Chen C, et al. The evolutionarily conserved zinc finger motif in the largest subunit of human replication protein A is required for DNA replication and mismatch repair but not for nucleotide excision repair. J Biol Chem. 1998;273:1453–61.
48. Gu L, Hong Y, McCulloch S, et al. ATP-dependent interaction of human mismatch repair proteins and dual role of PCNA in mismatch repair. Nucleic Acids Res. 1998;26:1173–8.
49. Zhang Y, Yuan F, Presnell SR, et al. Reconstitution of 5′-directed human mismatch repair in a purified system. Cell. 2005;122:693–705.
50. Genschel J, Littman SJ, Drummond JT, et al. Isolation of MutSbeta from human cells and comparison of the mismatch repair specificities of MutSbeta and MutSalpha. J Biol Chem. 1998;273(31):19895–901.
51. Iyer RR, Pluciennik A, Genschel J, et al. MutLalpha and proliferating cell nuclear antigen share binding sites on MutSbeta. J Biol Chem. 2010;285(15):11730–9.
52. Plotz G, Raedle J, Brieger A, et al. N-terminus of hMLH1 confers interaction of hMutLalpha and hMutLbeta with hMutSalpha. Nucleic Acids Res. 2003;31(12):3217–26.
53. Dahal BK, Kadyrova LY, Delfino KR, et al. Involvement of DNA mismatch repair in the maintenance of heterochromatic DNA stability in *Saccharomyces cerevisiae*. PLoS Genet. 2017;13(10):e1007074.
54. Villahermosa D, Christensen O, Knapp K, et al. Schizosaccharomyces pombe MutSα and MutLα maintain stability of tetra-nucleotide repeats and Msh3 of hepta-nucleotide repeats. G3 (Bethesda). 2017;7(5):1463–73.
55. Prolla TA, Baker SM, Harris AC, et al. Tumour susceptibility and spontaneous mutation in mice deficient in Mlh1, Pms1 and Pms2 DNA mismatch repair. Nat Genet. 1998;18(3):276–9.
56. Jäger AC, Rasmussen M, Bisgaard HC, et al. HNPCC mutations in the human DNA mismatch repair gene hMLH1 influence assembly of hMutLalpha and hMLH1-hEXO1 complexes. Oncogene. 2001;20(27):3590–5.

57. Cannavo E, Marra G, Sabates-Bellver J, et al. Expression of the MutL homologue hMLH3 in human cells and its role in DNA mismatch repair. Cancer Res. 2005;65(23):10759–66.
58. Kadyrov FA, Dzantiev L, Constantin N, et al. Endonucleolytic function of MutLalpha in human mismatch repair. Cell. 2006;126(2):297–308.
59. Peng M, Litman R, Xie J, Sharma S, Brosh RM Jr, Cantor SB. The FANCJ/MutLalpha interaction is required for correction of the cross-link response in FA-J cells. EMBO J. 2007;26(13):3238–49.
60. Pluciennik A, Dzantiev L, Iyer RR, et al. PCNA function in the activation and strand direction of MutLα endonuclease in mismatch repair. Proc Natl Acad Sci U S A. 2010;107(37):16066–71.
61. Kunkel TA, Erie DA. DNA mismatch repair. Annu Rev Biochem. 2005;74:681–710.
62. Li GM. Mechanisms and functions of DNA mismatch repair. Cell Res. 2008;18(1):85–98.
63. Kunkel TA, Erie DA. Eukaryotic mismatch repair in relation to DNA replication. Annu Rev Genet. 2015;49:291–313.
64. Marti TM, Kunz C, Fleck O. DNA mismatch repair and mutation avoidance pathways. J Cell Physiol. 2002;191(1):28–41.
65. Friedberg EC. DNA damage and repair. Nature. 2003;421(6921):436–40.
66. Martin SA, Lord CJ, Ashworth A. Therapeutic targeting of the DNA mismatch repair pathway. Clin Cancer Res. 2010;16(21):5107–13.
67. Boland CR, Goel A. Microsatellite instability in colorectal cancer. Gastroenterology. 2010;138(6):2073–87.
68. Fishel R. Mismatch repair. J Biol Chem. 2015;290(44):26395–403.
69. Groothuizen FS, Sixma TK. The conserved molecular machinery in DNA mismatch repair enzyme structures. DNA Repair (Amst). 2016;38:14–23.
70. Hingorani MM. Mismatch binding, ADP-ATP exchange and intramolecular signaling during mismatch repair. DNA Repair (Amst). 2016;38:24–31.
71. Kadyrova LY, Kadyrov FA. Endonuclease activities of MutLα and its homologs in DNA mismatch repair. DNA Repair (Amst). 2016;38:42–9.
72. Peltomäki P. update on Lynch syndrome genomics. Familial Cancer. 2016;15:385–93.
73. Liu D, Keijzers G, Rasmussen LJ. DNA mismatch repair and its many roles in eukaryotic cells. Mutat Res. 2017;773:174–87.
74. Lee JB, Cho WK, Park J, et al. Single-molecule views of MutS on mismatched DNA. DNA Repair (Amst). 2014;20:82–93.
75. Plotz G, Raedle J, Brieger A, et al. hMutSalpha forms an ATP-dependent complex with hMutLalpha and hMutLbeta on DNA. Nucleic Acids Res. 2002;30(3):711–8.
76. Plotz G, Piiper A, Wormek M, et al. Analysis of the human MutLalpha.MutSalpha complex. Biochem Biophys Res Commun. 2006;340(3):852–9.
77. Friedhoff P, Li P, Gotthardt J. Protein-protein interactions in DNA mismatch repair. DNA Repair (Amst). 2016;38:50–7.
78. Jeon Y, Kim D, Martin-Lopez JV, et al. Dynamic control of strand excision during human DNA mismatch repair. Proc Natl Acad Sci U S A. 2016;113(12):3281–6.
79. Fishel R. Mismatch repair, molecular switches, and signal transduction. Genes Dev. 1998;12(14):2096–101.
80. Ban C, Junop M, Yang W. Transformation of MutL by ATP binding and hydrolysis: a switch in DNA mismatch repair. Cell. 1999;97(1):85–97.
81. Spampinato C, Modrich P. The MutL ATPase is required for mismatch repair. J Biol Chem. 2000;275(13):9863–9.
82. Lamers MH, Winterwerp HH, Sixma TK. The alternating ATPase domains of MutS control DNA mismatch repair. ENBO J. 2003;22(3):746–56.
83. Kolodner RD, Marsischky GT. Eukaryotic DNA mismatch repair. Curr Opin Genet Dev. 1999;9(1):89–96.
84. Peltomäki P. Deficient DNA mismatch repair: a common etiologic factor for colon cancer. Hum Mol Genet. 2001;10(7):735–40.

85. Bellacosa A. Functional interactions and signaling properties of mammalian DNA mismatch repair proteins. Cell Death Differ. 2001;8(11):1076–92.
86. Scmidt MHM, Pearson CE. Disease associated repeat instability and mismatch repair. DNA Repair (Amst). 2016;38:117–26.
87. Campregher C, Schmid G, Ferk F, et al. MSH3-deficiency initiates EMAST without oncogenic transformation of human colon epithelial cells. PLoS One. 2012;7(11):e50541. https://doi.org/10.1371/journal.pone.0050541.
88. Tseng-Rogenski SS, Chung H, Wilk M, et al. Oxidative stress induces nuclear-to-cytosol shift of hMSH3, a potential mechanism for EMAST in colorectal cancer cells. PLoS One. 2012;7(11):e50616. https://doi.org/10.1371/journal.pone.0050616.
89. Watson MMC, Berg M, Søreide K. Prevalence and implications of elevated microsatellite alterations at selected tetranucleotides in cancer. Br J Cancer. 2014;111(5):823–7.
90. Carethers JM, Koi M, Tseng-Rogenski SS. EMAST is a form of microsatellite instability that is initiated by inflammation and modulates colorectal cancer progression. Genes (Basel). 2015;6(2):185–205.
91. Venderbosch S, van Lent-van Vliet S, de Haan AF, et al. EMAST is associated with a poor prognosis in microsatellite instable metastatic colorectal cancer. PLoS One. 2015;10(4):e0124538. https://doi.org/10.1371/journal.pone.0124538.
92. Dollé E, Theise ND, Schmelzer E, et al. EpCAM and the biology of hepatic stem/progenitor cells. Am J Physiol Gastrointest Liver Physiol. 2015;308:*G233*–50.
93. Huang L, Yang Y, Yang F, et al. Functions of EpCAM in physiological processes and diseases. Int J Mol Med. 2018;42(4):1771–85.
94. Kovacs ME, Papp J, Szentirmay Z, et al. Deletions removing the last exon of TACSTD1 constitute a distinct class of mutations predisposing to Lynch syndrome. Hum Mutat. 2009;30(2):197–203.
95. Reifen RM, Cutz E, Griffiths AM, et al. Tufting enteropathy: a newly recognized clinicopathological entity associated with refractory diarrhea in infants. J Pediatr Gastroenterol Nutr. 1994;18(3):379–85.
96. Goulet O, Salomon J, Ruemmele F, et al. Intestinal epithelial dysplasia (tufting enteropathy). Orphanet J Rare Dis. 2007;2(1):20.
97. Sivagnanam M, Mueller JL, Lee H, et al. Identification of EpCAM as the gene for congenital tufting enteropathy. Gastroenterology. 2008;135(2):429–37.
98. Pathak SJ, Mueller JL, Okamoto K, et al. EPCAM mutation update: variants associated with congenital tufting enteropathy and Lynch syndrome. Hum Mutat. 2019;40(2):142–61.
99. Wimmer K, Kratz CP, Vasen HFA, et al. Diagnostic criteria for constitutional mismatch repair deficiency syndrome: suggestions of the European consortium 'care for CMMRD' (C4CMMRD). J Med Genet. 2014;51(6):355–65.
100. Ricciardone MD, Ozçelik T, Cevher B, et al. Human MLH1 deficiency predisposes to hematological malignancy and neurofibromatosis type 1. Cancer Res. 1999;59(2):290–3.
101. Wang Q, Lasset C, Desseigne F, et al. Neurofibromatosis and early onset of cancers in hMLH1-deficient children. Cancer Res. 1999;59(2):294–7.
102. Turcot J, Despres JP, St Pierre F, et al. Malignant tumors of the central nervous system associated with familial polyposis of the colon: report of two cases. Dis Colon Rectum. 1959;2:465–8.
103. Hamilton SR, Liu B, Parsons RE, et al. The molecular basis of Turcot's syndrome. N Engl J Med. 1995;332(13):839–47.
104. Lavoine N, Colas C, Muleris M, et al. Constitutional mismatch repair deficiency syndrome: clinical description in a French cohort. J Med Genet. 2015;52(11):770–8.
105. Evaluation of Genomic Applications in Practice and Prevention (EGAPP) Working Group. Recommendations from the EGAPP Working Group: genetic testing strategies in newly diagnosed individuals with colorectal cancer aimed at reducing morbidity and mortality from Lynch syndrome in relatives. Genet Med. 2009;11(1):35–41.

106. Giardiello FM, Allen JI, Axilbund JE, et al. Guidelines on genetic evaluation and management of Lynch syndrome: a consensus statement by the US Multisociety Task Force on colorectal cancer. Am J Gastroenterol. 2014;109(8):1159–79.
107. Syngal S, Brand RE, Church JM, et al. ACG clinical guideline: genetic testing and management of hereditary gastrointestinal cancer syndromes. Am J Gastroenterol. 2015;110(2):223–62.
108. Boland CR, Thibodeau SN, Hamilton SR, et al. A National Cancer Institute Workshop on microsatellite instability for cancer detection and familial predisposition: development of international criteria for the determination of microsatellite instability in colorectal cancer. Cancer Res. 1998;58(22):5248–57.
109. Ionov Y, Peinado MA, Malkhosyan S, et al. Ubiquitous somatic mutations in simple repeated sequences reveal a new mechanism for colonic carcinogenesis. Nature. 1993;363(6429):558–61.
110. Peltomäki P, Aaltonen LA, Sistonen P, et al. Genetic mapping of a locus predisposing to human colorectal cancer. Nature. 1993;260:810–2.
111. Thibodeau SN, Bren G, Schaid D. Microsatellite instability in cancer of the proximal colon. Nature. 1993;260(5109):816–9.
112. Rodriguez-Bigas MA, Boland CR, Hamilton SR, et al. A National Cancer Institute Workshop on hereditary nonpolyposis colorectal cancer syndrome: meeting highlights and Bethesda guidelines. J Natl Cancer Inst. 1997;89(23):1758–62.
113. Leach FS, Polyak K, Burrell M, et al. Expression of the human mismatch repair gene hMSH2 in normal and neoplastic tissues. Cancer Res. 1996;56(2):235–40.
114. Thibodeau SN, French AJ, Roche PC, et al. Altered expression of hMSH2 and hMLH1 in tumors with microsatellite instability and genetic alterations in mismatch repair genes. Cancer Res. 1996;56(21):4836–40.
115. Hendriks Y, Franken P, Dierssen JW, et al. Conventional and tissue microarray immunohistochemical expression analysis of mismatch repair in hereditary colorectal tumors. Am J Pathol. 2003;162(2):469–77.
116. de Jong AE, van Puijenbroek M, Hendriks Y, et al. Microsatellite instability, immunohistochemistry, and additional PMS2 staining in suspected hereditary nonpolyposis colorectal cancer. Clin Cancer Res. 2004;10(39):972–80.
117. Lipkin SM, Wang V, Jacoby R, et al. MLH3: a DNA mismatch repair gene associated with mammalian microsatellite instability. Nat Genet. 2000;24(1):27–35.
118. Rigau V, Sebbagh N, Olschwang S, et al. Microsatellite instability in colorectal carcinoma. The comparison of immunohistochemistry and molecular biology suggests a role for hMSH6 [correction of hMLH6] immunostaining. Arch Pathol Lab Med. 2003;127(6):694–700.
119. Hampel H, Frankel WL, Martin E, et al. Screening for the Lynch syndrome (hereditary nonpolyposis colorectal cancer). N Engl J Med. 2005;352(18):1851–60.
120. Hendriks YMC, de Jong AE, Morreau H, et al. Diagnostic approach and management of Lynch syndrome (hereditary nonpolyposis colorectal carcinoma): a guide for clinicians. CA Cancer J Clin. 2006;56(4):213–25.
121. Snowsill T, Coelho H, Huxley N, et al. Molecular testing for Lynch syndrome in people with colorectal cancer: systematic reviews and economic evaluation. Health Technol Assess. 2017;21(51):1–238.
122. Jin M, Hampel H, Zhou X, et al. *BRAF* V600E mutation analysis simplifies the testing algorithm for Lynch Syndrome. Am J Clin Pathol. 2013;140(2):177–83.
123. Lagerstedt-Robinson K, Rohlin A, Aravidis C, et al. Mismatch repair gene mutation spectrum in the Swedish Lynch syndrome population. Oncol Rep. 2016;36(5):2823–35.
124. Lorans M, Dow E, Macrae FA, et al. Update on hereditary colorectal cancer: improving the clinical utility of multigene panel testing. Clin Colorectal Cancer. 2018;17(2):e293–305. https://doi.org/10.1016/j.clcc.2018.01.001.
125. Gallego CJ, Shirts BH, Bennette CS, et al. Next-generations sequencing panels for the diagnosis of colorectal cancer and polyposis syndromes: a cost-effectiveness analysis. J Clin Oncol. 2015;33(18):2084–91.

126. Espenschied CR, LaDuca H, Li S, et al. Multigene panel testing provides a new perspective on Lynch syndrome. J Clin Oncol. 2017;35(22):2568–75.
127. Yurgelun MB, Kulke MH, Fuchs CS, et al. Cancer susceptibility gene mutations in individuals with colorectal cancer. J Clin Oncol. 2017;35(10):1086–95.
128. Thompson BA, Spurdle AB, Plazzer JP, et al. Application of a 5-tiered scheme for standardized classification of 2,360 unique mismatch repair gene variants in the InSiGHT locus-specific database. Nat Genet. 2014;46(12):107–15.
129. Roberts ME, Jackson SA, Susswein LR, et al. *MSH6* and *PMS2* germ-line pathogenic variants implicated in Lynch syndrome are associated with breast cancer. Genet Med. 2018;20(10):1167–74.
130. Plazzer JP, Sijmons RH, Woods MO, et al. The InSiGHT database: utilizing 100 years of insights into Lynch syndrome. Familial Cancer. 2013;12(2):175–80.
131. Leach DR, Krummel MF, Allison JP. Enhancement of antitumor immunity by CTLA-4 blockade. Science. 1996;271(5256):1734–6.
132. Ishida Y, Agata Y, Shibahara K, Honjo T. Induced expression of PD-1, a novel member of the immunoglobulin gene superfamily, upon programmed cell death. EMBO J. 1992;11(11):3887–95.
133. Tivol EA, Borriello F, Schweitzer AN, et al. Loss of CTLA-4 leads to massive lymphoproliferation and fatal multiorgan tissue destruction, revealing a critical negative regulatory role of CTLA-4. Immunity. 1995;3(5):541–7.
134. Nishimura H, Nose M, Hiai H, et al. Development of lupus-like autoimmune diseases by disruption of the PD-1 gene encoding an ITIM motif-carrying immunoreceptor. Immunity. 1999;11(2):141–51.
135. Topalian SL, Hodi S, Brahmer JR, et al. Safety, activity, and immune correlates of anti-PD-1 antibody in cancer. N Engl J Med. 2012;366(26):2443–54.
136. Le DT, Uram JN, Wang H, et al. PD-1 blockade in tumors with mismatch-repair deficiency. N Engl J Med. 2015;372(26):2509–20.
137. Yarchoan M, Hopkins A, Jaffee EM, et al. Tumor mutational burden and response rate to PD-1 inhibition. N Engl J Med. 2018;377(25):2500–1.
138. Snyder A, Makarov V, Merghoub T, et al. Genetic basis for clinical response to CTLA-4 blockade in melanoma. N Engl J Med. 2014;371(23):2189–99.
139. Rizvi NA, Hellmann MD, Snyder A, et al. Cancer immunology. Mutational landscape determines sensitivity to PD-1blockade in non-small cell lung cancer. Science. 2015;348(6230):124–8.
140. Charmers ZR, Connelly CF, Fabrizio D, et al. Analysis of 100,000 human cancer genomes reveals the landscape of tumor mutational burden. Genome Med. 2017;9(1):34. https://doi.org/10.1186/s13073-017-0424-2.
141. Dudley JC, Lin MT, Le DT, et al. Microsatellite instability as a biomarker for PD-1 blockade. Clin Cancer Res. 2016;22(4):813–20.
142. Le DT, Durham JN, Smith KN, et al. Mismatch repair deficiency predicts response of solid tumors to PD-1 blockade. Science. 2017;357(6349):409–13.

Clinical Features of Lynch Syndrome

2

Kohji Tanakaya

Abstract

Lynch syndrome (LS) is one of the most common genetic cancer syndromes and accounts for 1–4% of all colorectal cancer cases. It is estimated that more than 100,000 individuals in Japan carry LS variants. This autosomal dominant disease is mainly caused by germline variants of mismatch repair genes (*MSH2*, *MLH1*, *MSH6*, *PMS2*) or *EPCAM*. Individuals with LS tend to develop with various types of tumors at a young age, such as colorectal cancer, endometrial cancer, and gastric cancer. The risk of developing LS-associated tumors may vary greatly depending on the population, gender of the carrier, and mismatch repair gene mutated. In this chapter, we discuss the clinical features of LS.

Keywords

Lynch syndrome · Mismatch repair genes · Colorectal cancer · Endometrial cancer · Gastric cancer · Ovarian cancer · Biliary tract cancer

2.1 Hereditary Colorectal Cancer

Cancer is a leading cause of death worldwide, accounting for an estimated 9.6 million deaths in 2018. Colorectal cancer (CRC) is the third-most common cancer, with 1.8 million new cases in 2018 [1]. In Japan, it is currently estimated that about 10% of men and 8% of women will be diagnosed with CRC during their lifetime [2].

K. Tanakaya (✉)
Department of Surgery, National Hospital Organization Iwakuni Clinical Center, Iwakuni, Yamaguchi, Japan
e-mail: tanakaya.kouji.tb@mail.hosp.go.jp

N. Tomita (ed.), *Lynch Syndrome*, https://doi.org/10.1007/978-981-15-6891-6_2

CRC is caused by multiple factors. Approximately 70–80% of CRC cases seem to be sporadic. In contrast, in the remaining 20–30% of CRC, the familial accumulation of CRC cases, known as familial CRC, is observed [3]. In approximately 5–10% of CRC cases, the causative genes have been identified, and these cases are referred to as hereditary CRC [4–6].

2.2 History

In 1895, Aldred Warthin, a pathologist of the University of Michigan, started his study on cancer fraternity. A young seamstress told him about her family that had shown an accumulation of cancer over several generations at an early age, including mainly gastric cancer (GC) and endometrial cancer (EC). Her family had migrated from Germany. Warthin reported this series as "family G" in 1913 [7]. Warthin suspected the existence of underlying hereditary factors in Family G. However, in that era, the influence of heredity factors on cancer susceptibility had not yet been recognized.

In 1966, Henry Lynch and Margery Shaw et al. reported two families—family N from Nebraska, and family M from Michigan. Lynch and Shaw had discovered the existence of genetic cancer syndromes with an autosomal dominant fashion [8].

In 1993, *MSH2*, one of the causative genes of LS, was first discovered. Three other mismatch repair (MMR) genes (*MLH1*, *MSH6*, *PMS2*), and *EPCAM* were subsequently also identified as causative genes for LS [9–11]. *EPCAM* is upstream adjacent to *MSH2*, and the germline deletion of the 3′ end of *EPCAM* causes *MSH2* silencing via methylation of the *MSH2* promoter region [11].

The role of DNA MMR function is to maintain genomic stability by correcting base mismatches and insertion–deletion mismatches that can arise during DNA replication. When the DNA MMR function is impaired, the sequence repeat number in simple repetitive sequences (microsatellites) is prone to changes. The altered number of repetitive sequences in microsatellites is termed microsatellite instability (MSI). LS-associated tumors with variants in MMR genes therefore commonly show a high frequency of MSI (MSI-H) [9, 12, 13].

2.3 Definition

LS is an autosomal dominant disease caused by a germline variant in one of the DNA MMR genes (*MLH1*, *MSH2*, *MSH6*, *PMS2*) or the *EPCAM* gene.

The term "Lynch syndrome" is often used synonymously with "hereditary nonpolyposis colorectal cancer (HNPCC)." However, some hold that LS refers to genetically confirmed patients and or families, while HNPCC refers to patients and families who clinically fulfill the Amsterdam I [14] or II [15] criteria (Tables 2.1 and 2.2) without a genetic diagnosis.

Table 2.1 Amsterdam criteria I

At least three relatives must have a colorectal cancer; all the following criteria should be met
1. One must be a first-degree relative of the other two
2. At least two successive generations must be affected
3. At least one should have been diagnosed before the age 50 years
4. Familial adenomatous polyposis should be excluded
5. Tumor diagnosis should be confirmed by histopathological examination

Table 2.2 Amsterdam criteria II

At least three relatives must have a Lynch syndrome-associated cancer (colorectal, endometrial, small bowel, ureter, or renal pelvic cancer); all of the following criteria should be met
1. One must be a first-degree relative of the other two
2. At least two successive generations must be affected
3. At least one should have been diagnosed before the age 50 years
4. Familial adenomatous polyposis should be excluded
5. Tumor diagnosis should be confirmed by histopathological examination

2.4 Prevalence

Estimates of the population prevalence of LS vary from 1:226 to 1:2000 [9, 10, 16]. LS accounts for 0.7–4% of all CRC cases [17–20] and 1–6% of all EC cases [9, 21]. The number of individuals with LS in Japan is estimated to be more than 100,000.

2.5 LS-Associated Cancer

Individuals with LS have a high risk for CRC, EC, GC, ovarian cancer (OC), pancreas cancer, renal pelvic/ureteral cancer, biliary tract cancer, brain tumors, sebaceous tumors, keratoacanthoma, and small intestinal cancer [22]. Recent reports show that breast cancer [23, 24], prostate cancer [25], and sarcoma [26, 27] are also LS-associated cancers. Not all individuals with LS will develop cancer. In other words, showing an incomplete penetrance. These risks vary depending on the population, gender of the carriers, and MMR gene mutated. The cumulative risk of cancer at 70 years of age is significantly higher in *MSH2* and *MLH1* variant carriers than in *MSH6* or *PMS2* variants (Table 2.3).

Table 2.3 Cumulative risk of Lynch syndrome-associated cancer at 70 years of age

Cancer (gene)		General population risk in the US [28] (Lifetime risk [29])	General population risk in Japan [2]	Lynch syndrome risk (%)	Average age at the diagnosis (years)	References
Colon		M:3.3%, F:3%	M: 3%, F: 2%			
(MLH1/MSH2)	M			22–74	27–60	[30–39]
	F			22–61		
(MSH6)	M			12–22	54–63	[31, 37–39]
	F			10–30		
(PMS2)	M			0–20	47–66	[38–40]
	F			0–15		
Endometrium		1.50%	1%			
(MLH1/MSH2)				14–54	48–62	[30, 31, 33, 35, 37–39, 41]
(MSH6)				16–71	53–54	[31, 37–39, 41, 42]
(PMS2)				13–26	49–50	[38, 39, 41]
Stomach		(0.80%)	M: 3%, F: 1%	5.8–13	49–55	[43–47]
Ovary		(1.20%)	1%	3.4–22	42–54	[37, 45, 46, 48–51]
Biliary tract				0.02–4	54–57	[37, 45, 49, 50]
Urinary tract				0.2–25	52–60	[37, 45, 46, 48–50]
Small bowel		(0.30%)		0.4–12	46–49	[37, 45, 46, 48, 49]
Skin				1–9	51–54	[52–54]
Brain/central nervous system		(0.60%)	M: 0.2%, F: 0.2%	1.2–3.7	50–55	[37, 46, 48, 49, 55]
Pancreas		(1.60%)	M: 0.6%, F: 0.4%	0.4–3.7	52–57	[33, 38, 56]

Since CRC and EC are the most common LS-associated cancers and develop at relatively early ages [57], their development often can be a clue for the diagnosis of LS. Traditionally, as the first step for the diagnosis of LS, clinical criteria such as the Amsterdam criteria II (Table 2.2) [15] or revised Bethesda guidelines (Table 2.4) [22] had been used for selecting individuals for further testing. However, screening by using these criteria or guidelines could miss more than one-fourth of LS cases [18]. Therefore, many experts recommend screening all patients with CRC using either MSI testing or immunohistochemistry (IHC) [9, 10, 12, 58].

Among *MSH2* and *MLH1* variant carriers, CRC shows the highest cumulative risk, followed by EC and other extracolonic cancers. With regard to extracolonic cancers, *MSH2* variants may be associated with higher risks than *MLH1* variants.

Table 2.4 The revised Bethesda guidelines for colorectal cancers for microsatellite instability testing

Tumors from patients with colorectal cancer (CRC) should be tested for MSI in the following situations
1. CRC diagnosed in a patient less than 50 years old
2. Presence of synchronous, metachronous colorectal, or other Lynch syndrome (LS)-associated tumors[a], regardless of the age
3. CRC with MSI-H histology[b] diagnosed in a patient less than 60 years old
4. CRC diagnosed in a patient with one or more first-degree relatives with a LS-associated tumor, with one of the cancers being diagnosed under the age of 50 years
5. CRC diagnosed in two or more first- or second-degree relatives with LS-associated tumors, regardless of the age

[a]LS-associated tumors include colorectal cancer, endometrial cancer, gastric cancer, small intestinal cancer, ovarian cancer, pancreatic cancer, renal pelvic/ureteral cancer, biliary tract cancer, brain tumors, sebaceous gland adenomas, and keratoacanthomas

[b]Tumor infiltrating lymphocytes, Crohn's-like lymphocytic reaction, mucinous/signet ring differentiation, or medullary growth pattern

Of note: the EC risk is higher than the CRC risk among female carriers of *MSH6* variants and may be higher than the CRC risk among female carriers of *PMS2* variants.

Marked differences in the disease phenotype are often observed both within and between families of LS [59, 60]. Although previous studies have suggested that the disease phenotype might be attributed to the effects of modifier genes, at present, no significant modifier genes have been identified in LS [61, 62].

2.6 CRC

The most common LS-associated cancer is CRC, which is characterized by an early age of onset, the occurrence of multiple tumors, and preferential development in the right colon.

CRC in LS develops through the adenoma-carcinoma sequence, just as in cases of sporadic CRC [59]. However, the progression from colon adenoma to cancer is faster in LS (<3 years) than in sporadic cases (10–15 years) [63]. With regard to the number of polyps, carriers of LS do not present clinically with polyposis, instead showing only a few adenomas.

The presence of deficiency of MMR (dMMR) in the tumor can be assessed by MSI testing or by IHC for loss of expression of MMR proteins. CRC in LS shows MSI-H at frequencies of 85–90% [58, 64, 65]. Therefore, CRC in LS often presents with the histological features of MSI-H CRC, which include the presence of tumor-infiltrating lymphocytes, a medullary growth pattern, mucinous/signet ring cell differentiation, and Crohn's-like lymphocytic reaction [22]. Ten to fifteen percent of all CRCs show MSI-H in Western countries [9, 65, 66], whereas, in Japan, 6–7% show MSI-H [16, 67, 68].

Sporadic CRC also shows MSI-H, largely due to epigenetic hypermethylation of the promoter region of the *MLH1* gene [22]. To rule out sporadic MSI-H CRC,

BRAF V600E testing can be used [9, 65, 66]. The *BRAF* V600E somatic variant is observed in approximately 40% of sporadic MSI-H CRC cases [69, 70] but rarely in LS. IHC for BRAF protein expression (clone VE1) can also be used to rule out sporadic MSI-H CRC [71].

The cumulative risk at 70 years old for developing CRC in variant carriers is reported to be up to 74% [30–39] depending on the gender and causative gene. Male variant carriers have a higher risk of CRC than female variant carriers. Furthermore, *MLH1* and *MSH2* variant carriers are suggested to have a higher risk for CRC and an earlier age of onset (27–60 years) [30–39] than *MSH6* (54–63 years) [31, 37–39] and *PMS2* variant carriers (47–66 years) [38–40].

Patients with CRC in LS show a better prognosis than those with sporadic CRC [39, 41, 72, 73]. This survival advantage has been attributed to immunological host defense mechanisms, such as an increased number of tumor-infiltrating lymphocytes.

2.7 EC

The second-most common LS-associated cancer is EC, which is characterized by an early age of onset [36] and a high prevalence of lower uterine segment (5.3–29%) [74, 75] and synchronous/metachronous OC [76]. The cumulative risk for EC in *MSH6* gene variant carriers is 16–71% [31, 37–39, 41, 42], which is equivalent to or higher than the risk for *MSH2*/*MLH1* gene variant carriers (14–54%) [30, 31, 33, 35, 37–39, 41]. The cumulative risk for EC in *PMS2* carriers is 0–24% [38, 39, 41], which is lower than in other carriers, including those with *MLH1*, *MSH2*, and *MSH6* gene variants. Patients with EC in LS show a *better* prognosis than sporadic EC, with an average 5-year survival rate of 93% [41].

2.8 GC

GC is the fourth-most common cancer and the second-most common cause of cancer death worldwide [43]. GC shows wide geographical variation in both incidence and mortality rates, possibly due to environmental, lifestyle, or genetic factors, including *Helicobacter pylori* infection, salt-preserved food consumption, dietary nitrite content, smoking and alcohol habits, obesity rates, radiation exposure, and Epstein-Barr virus infection [43]. Note that the cancer spectrum of LS in the family with LS first reported by Warthin included mainly GC and EC [7]. However, follow-up reports of this family showed that, in later generations, CRC was the most common tumor [8].

GC in LS is characterized by male dominance, an early age at onset, and the occurrence of multiple tumors. Regarding the pathological type of GC in LS, the intestinal type is predominant [44]. The cumulative risk of GC at 70 years of age in LS cases is 6–13% in Western countries [45–47, 77] and 24% in Japan (up to age 60 years) [78]. Due to the high frequency of death due to GC among patients with LS in Japan, the management of GC is as important as that of CRC and EC [79]. Patients with GC in LS show an average 5-year survival rate of 61% [41].

2.9 OC

OC in LS developes at an average age of 42-54 years [37, 45, 46, 48–51]. Regarding the histological subtype, endometrioid adenocarcinoma is predominant [51]. The cumulative risk of OC at 70 years of age in LS cases is 3.4–22% [37, 45, 46, 48–51]. Patients with OC in LS show a good prognosis with a 5-year survival rate of 83% [41].

2.10 Biliary Tract Cancer

Biliary tract cancers are *MLH1* variant-predominant [41]. Biliary tract cancer in LS develops at an average age of 54–57 years [37, 45, 49, 50]. The cumulative risk of biliary tract cancer at 70 years of age in LS cases is 0.02–4% [37, 45, 49, 50]. Biliary tract cancer has a high incidence in the general population in eastern Asia and is an aggressive malignancy with a poor prognosis. Patients with biliary tract cancer in LS also show a poor prognosis, with an average 5-year survival rate of 29% [41]. The biliary tract may become an important target organ of cancer surveillance strategies in Japan for patients with LS.

2.11 Urinary Tract Cancer

Urinary tract cancer in LS includes the upper urinary tract and urinary bladder. Urothelial cancers are *MSH2* variant-predominant [41, 80]. Urinary tract cancer in LS develops at an average age of 52–60 years [37, 45, 46, 48–50]. The cumulative risk of urinary tract cancer at 70 years of age in LS is 0.2–25% [37, 45, 46, 48–50]. Patients with urinary tract cancer in LS show a good prognosis with an average 5-year survival rate of 85% and 93% for cancers of the upper urinary tract and urinary bladder, respectively [41].

2.12 Small Bowel Cancer

Almost 50% of all cases of small bowel cancer in LS are located in the duodenum [9, 81]. Small bowel cancer in LS develops at an average age of 46–49 years [37, 45, 46, 48, 49]. The cumulative risk of small bowel cancer at 70 years of age in LS is 0.4–12% [37, 45, 46, 48, 49].

2.13 Skin Cancer

In 1981, Lynch et al. reported the first observation of the cutaneous features of Muir–Torre syndrome (MTS) in LS [82]. MTS is a disease characterized by synchronous/metachronous development of various LS-associated tumors, such as

CRC with sebaceous tumors (sebaceous adenoma, sebaceous epithelioma, or sebaceous carcinoma) and/or keratoacanthoma. Due to the presence of widespread *MSH2* founder variants, *MSH2* variants are common in MTS [83]. The cumulative risk of skin cancer at 70 years of age in LS is 1–9% [52–54].

2.14 Brain Tumor

The complication of CRC with a primary brain tumor is defined as Turcot syndrome (TS). TS is divided into two types: Type 1 and Type 2, which are secondary to either MMR gene variants or *APC* gene variants, respectively. The brain tumors in individuals with *APC* variants are typically medulloblastoma, whereas those with MMR variants are usually glioblastoma multiforme. Brain tumors are *MSH2* variant-predominant [41]. Although an immunohistochemical analysis of these brain tumors has shown the absence of the MMR protein corresponding to the gene variant in the germline, the frequency of MSI-H in brain tumors is very low (0% for the brain) [55]. The cumulative risk of brain tumor at 70 years of age in LS is 1–4% [37, 46, 48, 49, 55]. Patients with brain tumor in LS show a poor prognosis, with an average 5-year survival rate of 22% [41].

2.15 Pancreatic Cancer

Several studies suggested that pancreatic cancer is associated with LS [33, 38, 56]. Pancreatic cancer in LS is *MLH1* variant-predominant [41] and develops at an average age of 52–57 years with a cumulative risk at 70 years of age in LS of 0.4–3.7% [33, 38, 56]. Patients with pancreatic cancer in LS show a very poor prognosis, with an average 5-year survival rate of 0% [41].

References

1. International Agency for Research on Cancer World Health Organization. Globocan 2018. https://gco.iarc.fr/today/data/factsheets/populations/900-world-fact-sheets.pdf. Accessed Apr 2020.
2. Cancer Registry and Statistics. Cancer Information Service, National Cancer Center, Japan. https://ganjoho.jp/reg_stat/statistics/stat/summary.html [in Japanese]. Accessed Apr 2020.
3. Brandão C, Lage J. Management of patients with hereditary colorectal cancer syndromes. GE Port J Gastroenterol. 2015;22:204–12.
4. Underhill ML, Germansky KA, Yurgelun MB. Advances in hereditary colorectal and pancreatic cancers. Clin Ther. 2016;38:1600–21.
5. Yurgelun MB, Kulke MH, Fuchs CS, et al. Cancer susceptibility gene mutations in individuals with colorectal cancer. J Clin Oncol. 2017;35:1086–95.
6. Lynch HT, Shaw TG. Practical genetics of colorectal cancer. Chin Clin Oncol. 2013;2:12.
7. Warthin AS. Heredity with reference to carcinoma as shown by the study of the cases examined in the pathological laboratory of the University of Michigan, 1895–1913. Arch Int Med. 1913;12:546–55.

8. Lynch HT, Shaw MW, Magnuson CW, et al. Hereditary factors in cancer. study of two large midwestern kindreds. Arch Intern Med. 1966;117:206–12.
9. Kohlmann W, Gruber SB. Lynch syndrome. Gene Rev. 2004. https://www.ncbi.nlm.nih.gov/books/NBK1211/. Accessed Apr 2020.
10. The International Society for Gastrointestinal Hereditary Tumours (InSiGHT). Lynch syndrome. 2020. https://www.insight-grouporg/syndromes/lynch-syndrome/. Accessed Apr 2020.
11. Ligtenberg MJ, Kuiper RP, Chan TL, et al. Heritable somatic methylation and inactivation of MSH2 in families with Lynch syndrome due to deletion of the 3′ exons of TACSTD1. Nat Genet. 2009;41:112–7.
12. Ishida H, Yamaguchi T, Tanakaya K, et al. Japanese Society for Cancer of the Colon and Rectum (JSCCR) guidelines 2016 for the clinical practice of hereditary colorectal cancer (translated version). J Anus Rectum Colon (JARC). 2018. http://journal-arc.jp/pdf/002s10001.pdf. Accessed Apr 2020.
13. Thibodeau SN, Bren G, Schaid D. Microsatellite instability in cancer of the proximal colon. Science. 1993;260:816–9.
14. Vasen HF, Mecklin JP, Khan PM, et al. The International Collaborative Group on hereditary non-polyposis colorectal cancer (ICG-HNPCC). Dis Colon Rectum. 1991;34:424–5.
15. Vasen HF, Watson P, Mecklin JP, et al. New clinical criteria for hereditary nonpolyposis colorectal cancer (HNPCC, Lynch syndrome) proposed by the International Collaborative group on HNPCC. Gastroenterology. 1999;116:1453–6.
16. de la Chapelle A. The incidence of Lynch syndrome. Familial Cancer. 2005;4:233–7.
17. Chika N, Eguchi H, Kumamoto K, et al. Prevalence of LS and Lynch-like syndrome among patients with colorectal cancer in a Japanese hospital-based population. Jpn J Clin Oncol. 2017;47:108–17.
18. Hampel H, Frankel WL, Martin E, et al. Feasibility of screening for LS among patients with colorectal cancer. J Clin Oncol. 2008;26:5783–8.
19. Moreira L, Balaguer F, Lindor N, et al. Identification of Lynch syndrome among patients with colorectal cancer. JAMA. 2012;308:1555–65.
20. Peltomäki P. Update on Lynch syndrome genomics. Familial Cancer. 2016;15:385–93.
21. Wang A, McCracken J, Li Y, Xu L. The practice of universal screening for Lynch syndrome in newly diagnosed endometrial carcinoma. Health Sci Rep. 2018;1:e43.
22. Umar A, Boland CR, Terdiman JP, et al. Bethesda guidelines for hereditary nonpolyposis colorectal cancer (Lynch Syndrome) and microsatellite instability. J Natl Cancer Inst. 2004;96:261–8.
23. Walsh MD, Buchanan DD, Cummings MC, et al. Lynch syndrome–associated breast cancers: clinicopathologic characteristics of a case series from the colon cancer family registry. Clin Cancer Res. 2010;16:2214–24.
24. Win AK, Lindor NM, Jenkins MA. Risk of breast cancer in Lynch syndrome: a systematic review. Breast Cancer Res. 2013;15:R27.
25. Raymond VM, Mukherjee B, Wang F, et al. Elevated risk of prostate cancer among men with Lynch syndrome. J Clin Oncol. 2013;31:1713–8.
26. Hirata K, Kanemitsu S, Nakayama Y, et al. A novel germline mutation of MSH2 in a hereditary nonpolyposis colorectal cancer patient with liposarcoma. HNPCC registry and genetic testing project of the Japanese Society for Cancer of the Colon and Rectum (JSCCR). Am J Gastroenterol. 2006;101:193–6.
27. Nilbert M, Therkildsen C, Nissen A, et al. Sarcomas associated with hereditary nonpolyposis colorectal cancer: broad anatomical and morphological spectrum. Familial Cancer. 2009;8:209–13.
28. Siegel RL, Miller KD, Jemal A. Cancer statistics, 2020. CA Cancer J Clin. 2020;70:7–30. https://acsjournals.onlinelibrary.wiley.com/doi/full/10.3322/caac.21590
29. Howlader N, Noone AM, Krapcho M, et al. SEER cancer statistics review, 1975–2017. National Cancer Institute, Bethesda, MD. 2020. https://seer.cancer.gov/csr/1975_2017/. Based on November 2019 SEER data submission, posted to the SEER web site, April 2020.

30. Dunlop MG, Farrington SM, Carothers AD, et al. Cancer risk associated with germline DNA mismatch repair gene mutations. Hum Mol Genet. 1997;6:105–10.
31. Quehenberger F, Vasen HF, van Houwelingen HC. Risk of colorectal and endometrial cancer for carriers of mutations of the hMLH1 and hMSH2 gene: correction for ascertainment. J Med Genet. 2005;42:491–6.
32. Hampel H, Stephens JA, Pukkala E, et al. Cancer risk in hereditary nonpolyposis colorectal cancer syndrome: later age of onset. Gastroenterology. 2005;129:415–21.
33. Jenkins MA, Baglietto L, Dowty JG, et al. Cancer risks for mismatch repair gene mutation carriers: a population-based early onset case-family study. Clin Gastroenterol Hepatol. 2006;4:489–98.
34. Alarcon F, Lasset C, Carayol J, et al. Estimating cancer risk in HNPCC by the GRL method. Eur J Hum Genet. 2007;15:831–6.
35. Choi YH, Cotterchio M, McKeown-Eyssen G, et al. Penetrance of colorectal cancer among MLH1/MSH2 carriers participating in the colorectal cancer familial registry in Ontario. Hered Cancer Clin Pract. 2009;23:14.
36. Bonadona V, Bonaïti B, Olschwang S, et al. Cancer risks associated with germline mutations in MLH1, MSH2, and MSH6 genes in Lynch syndrome. JAMA. 2011;305:2304–10.
37. Baglietto L, Lindor NM, Dowty JG, et al. Risks of Lynch syndrome cancers for MSH6 mutation carriers. J Natl Cancer Inst. 2010;102:193–201.
38. Møller P, Seppälä T, Bernstein I, et al. Cancer incidence and survival in Lynch syndrome patients receiving colonoscopic and gynaecological surveillance: first report from the prospective Lynch syndrome database. Gut. 2017;66:464–72.
39. Dominguez-Valentin M, Sampson JR, Seppälä TT, et al. Cancer risks by gene, age, and gender in 6350 carriers of pathogenic mismatch repair variants: findings from the Prospective Lynch Syndrome Database. Genet Med. 2019. https://doi.org/10.1038/s41436-0190596-9. Accessed Apr 2020.
40. Senter L, Clendenning M, Sotamaa K, et al. The clinical phenotype of Lynch syndrome due to germ-line PMS2 mutations. Gastroenterology. 2008;135:419–28.
41. Møller P, Seppälä TT, Bernstein I, et al. Cancer risk and survival in path_MMR carriers by gene and gender up to 75 years of age: a report from the Prospective Lynch Syndrome. Gut. 2018;67:1306–16.
42. Hendriks Y, Wagner A, Morreau H, et al. Cancer risk in hereditary nonpolyposis colorectal cancer due to MSH6 mutations: impact on counseling and surveillance. Gastroenterology. 2004;127:17–25.
43. Sitarz R, Skierucha M, Mielko J, et al. Gastric cancer: epidemiology, prevention, classification, and treatment. Cancer Manag Res. 2018;7:239–48.
44. Aarnio M, Salovaara R, Aaltonen LA, et al. Features of gastric cancer in hereditary nonpolyposis colorectal cancer syndrome. Int J Cancer. 1997;21:551–5.
45. Engel C, Loeffler M, Steinke V, et al. Risks of less common cancers in proven mutation carriers with Lynch syndrome. J Clin Oncol. 2012;30:4409–15.
46. Watson P, Vasen HF, Mecklin JP, et al. The risk of extra-colonic, extra-endometrial cancer in the Lynch syndrome. Int J Cancer. 2008;123:444–9.
47. Capelle LG, Van Grieken NC, Lingsma HF, et al. Risk and epidemiological time trends of gastric cancer in Lynch syndrome carriers in the Netherlands. Gastroenterology. 2010;138:487–92.
48. Vasen H, Stormorken A, Menko F, et al. MSH2 mutation carriers are at higher risk of cancer than MLH1 mutation carriers: a study of hereditary nonpolyposis colorectal cancer families. J Clin Oncol. 2001;19:4074–80.
49. Barrow E, Robinson L, Alduaij W, et al. Cumulative lifetime incidence of extra colonic cancers in Lynch syndrome: a report of 121 families with proven mutations. Clin Genet. 2009;75:141–9.
50. Aarnio M, Sankila R, Pukkala E, et al. Cancer risk in mutation carriers of DNA-mismatch-repair genes. Int J Cancer. 1999;81:214–8.
51. Ryan NAJ, Evans DG, Green K, et al. Pathological features and clinical behavior of Lynchsyndrome-associatedovariancancer. Gynecol Oncol. 2017;144:491–5.

52. Ponti G, Losi L, Pedroni M, et al. Value of MLH1 and MSH2 mutations in the appearance of Muir–Torre syndrome phenotype in HNPCC patients presenting sebaceous gland tumors or keratoacanthomas. J Invest Dermatol. 2006;126:2302–7.
53. Schwartz RA, Torre DP. The Muir-Torre syndrome: a 25-year retrospect. J Am Acad Dermatol. 1995;33:90–104.
54. South CD, Hampel H, Comeras I, et al. The frequency of Muir-Torre syndrome among Lynch syndrome families. J Natl Cancer Inst. 2008;100:277–81.
55. Gylling A, Nieminen TT, Abdel-Rahman WM. Differential cancer predisposition in Lynch syndrome: insights from molecular analysis of brain and urinary tract tumors. Carcinogenesis. 2008;29:1351–9.
56. Kastrinos F, Mukherjee B, Tayob N, et al. Risk of pancreatic cancer in families with Lynch syndrome. JAMA. 2009;302:1790–5.
57. Ryan N, Morris J, Green K, et al. Association of mismatch repair mutation with age at cancer onset in Lynch syndrome: implications for stratified surveillance strategies. JAMA Oncol. 2017;3:1702–6.
58. Evaluation of Genomic Applications in Practice and Prevention (EGAPP) Working Group. Recommendations from the EGAPP Working Group: genetic testing strategies in newly diagnosed individuals with colorectal cancer aimed at reducing morbidity and mortality from Lynch syndrome in relatives. Genet Med. 2009;11:35–41.
59. Lynch HT, Smyrk TC, Watson P, et al. Genetics, natural history, tumor spectrum, and pathology of hereditary nonpolyposis colorectal cancer: an updated review. Gastroenterology. 1993;104:1535–49.
60. Talseth-Palmer BA, Wijnen JT, Grice DM, et al. Genetic modifiers of cancer risk in Lynch syndrome: a review. Fam Cancer. 2013;12:207–16.
61. Win AK, Hopper JL, Buchanan DD, et al. Are the common genetic variants associated with colorectal cancer risk for DNA mismatch repair gene mutation carriers? Eur J Cancer. 2013;49:1578–87.
62. Donald N, Malik S, McGuire JL, et al. The association of low penetrance genetic risk modifiers with colorectal cancer in lynch syndrome patients: a systematic review and meta-analysis. Familial Cancer. 2018;17:43–52.
63. Vasen HF, Nagengast FM, Khan PM. Interval cancers in hereditary non-polyposis colorectal cancer (Lynch syndrome). Lancet. 1995;345:1183–4.
64. Aaltonen LA, Peltomaki P, Mecklin JP, et al. Replication errors in benign and malignant tumors from hereditary nonpolyposis colorectal cancer patients. Cancer Res. 1994;54: 1645–8.
65. National Comprehensive Cancer Network. NCCN clinical practice guidelines in oncology (NCCN guidelines). Genetic/familial high-risk assessment: colorectal version 3.2019. Available via DIALOG http://www.nccn.org. Accessed Apr 2020.
66. Giardiello FM, Allen JI, Axilbund JE, et al. Guidelines on genetic evaluation and management of Lynch syndrome: a consensus statement by the US Multi-Society Task Force on colorectal cancer. Gastroenterology. 2014;147:502–26.
67. Ishikubo T, Nishimura Y, Yamaguchi K, et al. The clinical features of rectal cancers with high-frequency microsatellite instability (MSI-H) in Japanese males. Cancer Lett. 2004;216:55–62.
68. Asaka S, Arai Y, Nishimura Y, et al. Microsatellite instability-low colorectal cancer acquires a KRAS mutation during the progression from Dukes' A to Dukes' B. Carcinogenesis. 2009;30:494–9.
69. Koinuma K, Shitoh K, Miyakura Y, et al. Mutations of BRAF are associated with extensive hMLH1 promoter methylation in sporadic colorectal carcinomas. Int J Cancer. 2004;108:237–42.
70. McGivern A, Wynter CV, Whitehall VL, et al. Promoter hypermethylation frequency and BRAF mutations distinguish hereditary non-polyposis colon cancer from sporadic MSI-H colon cancer. Familial Cancer. 2004;3:101–10.
71. Long GV, Wilmott JS, Capper D, et al. Immunohistochemistry is highly sensitive and specific for the detection of V600E BRAF mutation in melanoma. Am J Surg Pathol. 2013;37:61–5.

72. Sankila R, Aaltonen LA, Järvinen HJ, et al. Better survival rates in patients with MLH1-associated hereditary colorectal cancer. Gastroenterology. 1996;110:682–7.
73. Stigliano V, Assisi D, Cosimelli M, et al. Survival of hereditary non-polyposis colorectal cancer patients compared with sporadic colorectal cancer patients. J Exp Clin Cancer Res. 2008;19:S39.
74. Ryan P, Mulligan AM, Aronson M, et al. Comparison of clinical schemas and morphologic features in predicting Lynch syndrome in mutation-positive patients with endometrial cancer encountered in the context of familial gastrointestinal cancer registries. Cancer. 2012;118:681–8.
75. Westin SN, Lacour RA, Urbauer DL, et al. Carcinoma of the lower uterine segment: a newly described association with Lynch syndrome. J Clin Oncol. 2008;26:5965–71.
76. Soliman PT, Broaddus RR, Schmeler KM, et al. Women with synchronous primary cancers of the endometrium and ovary: do they have Lynch syndrome? J Clin Oncol. 2005;23:9344–50.
77. Dowty JG, Win AK, Buchanan DD, et al. Cancer risks for MLH1 and MSH2 mutation carriers. Hum Mutat. 2013;34:490–7.
78. Yamaguchi T, Furukawa Y, Nakamura Y, et al. Comparison of clinical features between suspected familial colorectal cancer type X and LS in Japanese patients with colorec- tal cancer: a cross-sectional study conducted by the Japanese Society for Cancer of the Colon and Rectum. Jpn J Clin Oncol. 2014;45:153–9.
79. Tanakaya K, Yamaguchi T, Ishikawa H, et al. Causes of cancer death among first-degree relatives in Japanese families with Lynch syndrome; for HNPCC Registry and Genetic Testing Project of the Japanese Society for Cancer of the Colon and Rectum. Anticancer Res. 2016;36:1985–9.
80. Van der Post R, Kiemeney L, Ligtenberg M, et al. Risk of urothelial bladder cancer in Lynch syndrome is increased, in particular among MSH2 mutation carriers. J Med Genet. 2010;47:464–70.
81. Schulmann K, Brasch FE, Kunstmann E, et al. HNPCC-associated small bowel cancer: clinical and molecular characteristics. Gastroenterology. 2005;128:590–9.
82. Lynch HT, Lynch PM, Pester J, et al. The cancer family syndrome. Rare cutaneous phenotypic linkage of Torre's syndrome. Arch Intern Med. 1981;141:607–11.
83. Ponti G, Manfredini M, Tomasi A, et al. Muir-Torre syndrome and founder mismatch repair gene mutations: a long gone historical genetic challenge. Gene. 2016;10:127–32.

Pathology of Lynch Syndrome-Associated Tumors

3

Harumi Saeki and Okio Hino

Abstract

Lynch syndrome is caused by the DNA mismatch repair (MMR) genes, MLH1, MSH2, PMS2, MSH6, and EPCAM. Though the proteins encoded by these genes are stained by immunohistochemistry, and loss of the proteins can be recognized visually, the carcinoma lesions arising in Lynch syndrome have some characteristic histological features in hematoxylin-eosin (H&E) staining. Most of the Lynch syndrome carcinomas are Microsatellite Instability-High (MSI-High), and the histological findings are similar to those of the MSI-High carcinoma. In the revised Bethesda Guidelines, the features of colorectal cancer with MSI-High include the presence of tumor infiltrating lymphocytes (TILs), a Crohn's-like lymphocytic reaction, mucinous/signet-ring differentiation, or a medullary growth pattern. Other types of carcinoma in Lynch syndrome also show characteristic histology. In order to allow detection of the carcinomas in Lynch syndrome or Lynch-like syndrome without immunohistochemistry and molecular biological examinations, the histological characteristics of these carcinomas should be broadly understood.

Keywords

Lynch syndrome · MSI-High · Tumor infiltrating lymphocytes (TILs) · Crohn's-like lymphocytic reaction · Mucinous differentiation · Medullary growth pattern

H. Saeki
Department of Pathology and Oncology, Juntendo University Faculty of Medicine, Tokyo, Japan

Department of Human Pathology, Juntendo University Faculty of Medicine, Tokyo, Japan
e-mail: haru-s@juntendo.ac.jp

O. Hino (✉)
Department of Pathology and Oncology, Juntendo University Faculty of Medicine, Tokyo, Japan
e-mail: ohino@juntendo.ac.jp

N. Tomita (ed.), *Lynch Syndrome*, https://doi.org/10.1007/978-981-15-6891-6_3

3.1 Introduction

Lynch syndrome is caused by the DNA mismatch repair (MMR) genes, MLH1, MSH2, PMS2, MSH6, and EPCAM. It is possible to detect a loss of the MMR proteins by immunohistochemistry for MLH1, MSH2, PMS2, and MSH6, and pathologists can see some histological characteristics that correlate with hereditary cancer and predict those relationships. Therefore, it is important to know what kind of histological findings should be expected in specimens from patients with Lynch syndrome.

Most carcinomas arising in Lynch syndrome are Microsatellite Instability-High (MSI-High). Although the clinical futures differ for individuals with sporadic MSI-High carcinoma and those with Lynch syndrome carcinoma, the histological findings are similar [1]. Therefore, the histological characteristics of MSI-High carcinoma are those of the carcinomas arising in Lynch syndrome. The revised Bethesda Guidelines are widely used as the standard for assessment of Lynch syndrome [2].

3.2 Colorectal Cancer

In the revised Bethesda Guidelines, the features of colorectal cancer with the MSI-High include the presence of tumor infiltrating lymphocytes (TILs), a Crohn's-like lymphocytic reaction, mucinous/signet-ring differentiation, or medullary growth pattern [2].

3.2.1 Tumor Infiltrating Lymphocytes (TILs)

TILs are small round lymphocytes in the tumor epithelium associated with a peritumoral, stromal lymphocytic, or inflammatory infiltrate [3]. When TILs are evaluated histologically, intraepithelial lymphocytes, not peritumoral lymphocytes, should be counted as TILs (Fig. 3.1a, b). TILs consist of T cells, especially CD3-positive cells. We can see a bunch of infiltrating lymphocytes in the nest of tumor cells in hematoxylin-eosin (H&E) stains, and we can stain for T cell markers such as CD3 by immunohistochemistry. Some objective evaluation criteria for TILs have been reported and are used. In one method, MSI-High tumors were selected with a sensitivity of 75% by a count of more than 40 CD3-positive cells per 0.94 mm^2, and the specificity of the method was 67% [3].

3.2.2 Crohn's-Like Lymphocytic Reaction

A Crohn's-like lymphocytic reaction is defined as the presence of lymphoid follicles with or without germinal centers at the tumor's leading edge [3]. This means that the presence of existing lymphoid follicles in the mucosa or subserosa should

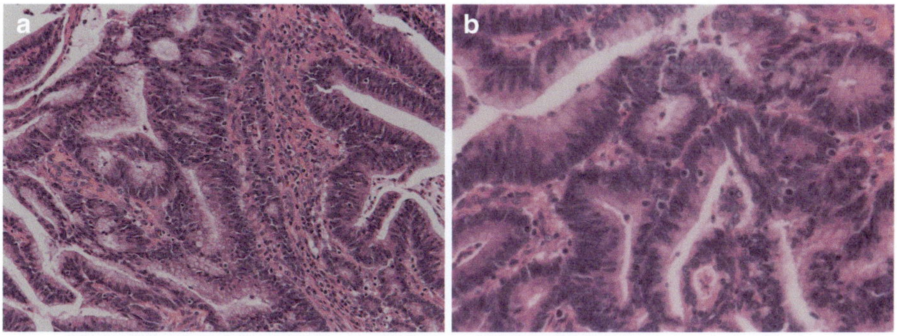

Fig. 3.1 Tumor infiltrating lymphocytes (TILs) [(**a**) Low power, (**b**) High power]. (**a**) Intraepithelial lymphocytes that are located among the epithelial cells are counted as TILs. (**b**) These lymphocytes have halos around them

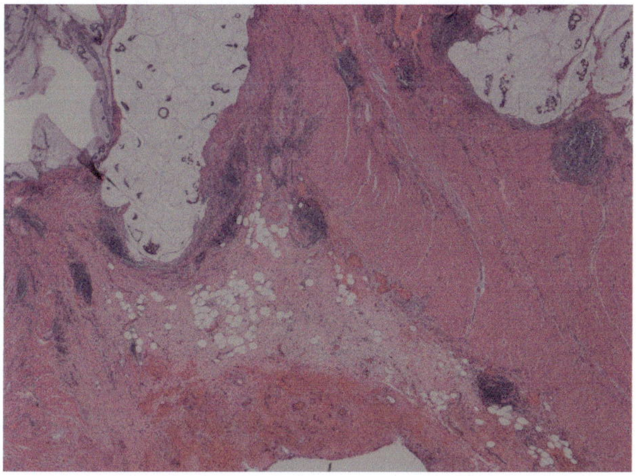

Fig. 3.2 Crohn's-like lymphocytic reaction: Lymphoid follicles with or without germinal centers at the tumor's leading edge

not be recognized as a Crohn's-like lymphocytic reaction (Fig. 3.2). Jenkins et al. scored a Crohn's-like lymphocytic reaction when at least four nodular lymphoid aggregates were counted in a low-power field beyond the advancing edge of the tumor [4].

3.2.3 Mucinous/Signet-Ring Differentiation

Mucinous carcinoma or signet-ring cell carcinoma is frequently found in the colorectal cancer arising in Lynch syndrome. Although various definitions of mucinous/signet-ring cell carcinoma are used, it is commonly accepted that the carcinoma should include at least 50% of the mucinous/signet-ring cell component [4]. In the WHO classification, mucinous carcinoma is defined as a lesion composed of pools of extracellular mucin [5] (Fig. 3.3). Signet-ring cell carcinoma in colorectal

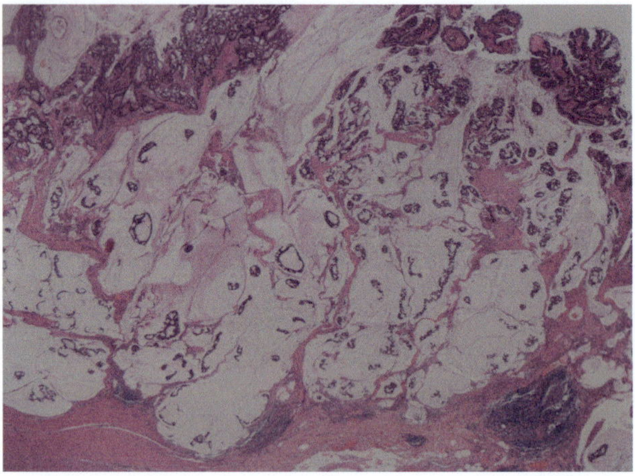

Fig. 3.3 Mucinous carcinoma. This lesion is composed of pools of extracellular mucin, and neoplastic cells float on the extracellular mucin

cancer is generally rare, its incidence is 1% or lower in previous reports regardless of hereditary cancer [6]. Mucinous carcinoma with >50% of the tumor including a mucinous histology component was identified in approximately 15% of MSI-High adenocarcinomas [1].

3.2.4 Medullary Growth Pattern

Medullary carcinoma also has many diagnostic criteria. Medullary carcinoma is defined as a tumor composed of masses of cells circumscribed by a margin and containing a marked lymphocytic infiltrate that is both peritumoral and intratumoral [4]. Most of the nuclei are small, and the cytoplasm is eosinophilic. Poorly differentiated or undifferentiated cells comprise a high percentage of medullary carcinoma cells.

Four histological endpoints in the revised Bethesda Guidelines are characterized as the histological characteristics of MSI-High carcinoma. Among them, mucinous carcinoma or poorly differentiated carcinoma, and TILs are especially useful to identify MSI-High carcinoma in histology [4].

MSI-High colorectal cancer is related to the *BRAF* mutation [7], and a tumor that has lost the MLH1 protein and shows the *BRAF* mutation is considered a sporadic colorectal cancer [8]. Regarding precursor lesions, although Lynch syndrome is classified as a non-polyposis syndrome, so as to be distinguished from Familial adenomatous polyposis, clinical data have shown that 40.7% of patients with a germline mutation in one of the four mismatch repair genes had one or more adenomas, and 4% of all patients had 10 or more cumulative adenomas [9]. It has been suggested that MSI-High colorectal cancer arising in Lynch syndrome is associated with adenoma and that adenoma is the precursor lesion for carcinoma in Lynch syndrome, but this suggested association is still unclear [10]. On the other hand, sessile serrated adenoma/polyp (SSA/P) is the precursor lesion for sporadic MSI-High colorectal cancer [11].

3.3 Endometrial Cancer

Endometrial cancer is the second most common cancer in Lynch syndrome. It has been suggested that endometrial cancer related to Lynch syndrome has various histological forms and no specific morphology: undifferentiated carcinoma, mucinous component, and rhabdoid cells with TILs or peritumoral lymphocyte invasion have all been observed. And 10–15% of endometrial cancers in Lynch syndrome arise in the lower uterine segment [12]. Endometrioid carcinoma is the most common histological type, but endometrial carcinoma arising in Lynch syndrome show a wide spectrum of histologic subtypes [12]. Tumors with loss of MMR proteins in immunohistochemistry frequently show undifferentiated or dedifferentiated histology and show a trend toward higher FIGO grades [13]. However, the predictive value of these findings to identify MMR mutations in the germline is uncertain [13]. The histology of undifferentiated or dedifferentiated endometrioid carcinoma is associated with MSI [14]. As with colorectal cancer, TILs, which are lymphocytes located within the nest of tumor cells or glands, and prominent peritumoral lymphocytes are linked to MSI in endometrial cancer [12] (Fig. 3.4a, b).

Sporadic and typical endometrial cancers in young patients are related to estrogen excess and the morphology is well differentiated type, but MMR defect-associated endometrial cancers have low estrogen receptor (ER)/progesterone receptor (PR) expression [13]. Whereas, other study has reported that ER expression showed no significant correlations with MSI status [15]. Higher FIGO grades or stages and lower ER/PR expression frequently are closely linked and coexist and are associated with a poor prognosis [13].

Some cases related to Lynch syndrome have no characteristics, as mentioned above, or do not satisfy clinical criteria such as the Amsterdam II criteria and the revised Bethesda Guidelines. Universal screening of patients with colorectal cancer to identify patients with Lynch syndrome by immunohistochemistry for the four MMR proteins is recommended. However, universal screening of patients with endometrial cancer is not performed widely [16]. Although the Society of

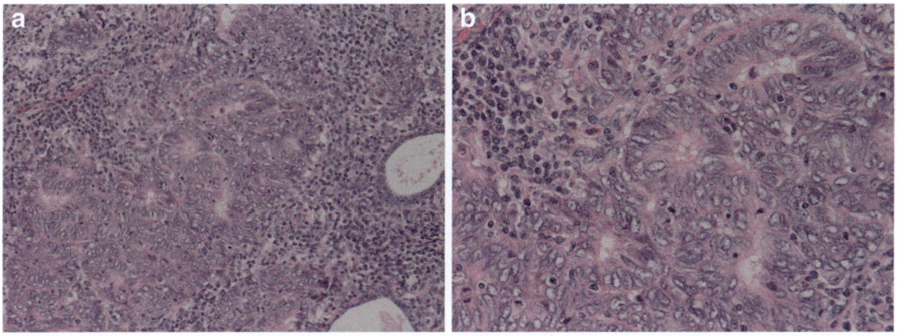

Fig. 3.4 Endometrial carcinoma [(**a**) Low power, (**b**) High power]. (**a**) MSI-High endometrial carcinoma. This is Endometrioid carcinoma, Grade 1. (**b**) TILs and peritumoral lymphocytes

Gynecologic Oncology recommends universal screening of patients with endometrial cancer, it is not broadly recommended [16].

3.4 Gastric Cancer

Gastric cancer is the third cancer in Lynch syndrome, and in males, it is the second most common cancer after colorectal cancer. The frequency of gastric cancer occurrence in Lynch syndrome mutation carriers is 1.6–18.1% [17–19]. However, the cumulative incidence of gastric cancer in Lynch syndrome patients is higher in East Asian countries than Western countries because of *Helicobacter pylori* infection [19]. Poorly differentiated carcinomas, including signet-ring cell carcinoma (diffuse-type gastric cancer), intestinal-type gastric cancer or mucinous carcinoma, have been suggested as the characteristic histological types of gastric cancer in Lynch syndrome [17, 20].

The intestinal-type gastric cancer is more prominent than the diffuse-type gastric cancer in Lynch syndrome, and especially in young patients [17]. The intestinal-type gastric cancer is closer related to *Helicobacter pylori* infection than is the diffuse-type gastric cancer [17]. Although the ratio of *Helicobacter pylori* infection in Western countries is lower than in East Asian countries, according to the American guidelines, patients with cancer risk caused by MMR mutations are monitored, and it is recommended that they undergo a screening esophagogastroduodenoscopy at age 30–35 and then every 2–3 years based on their individual risk factors [21].

3.5 Other Types of Carcinoma

Other types of cancer in Lynch syndrome, including ovarian, renal, pelvis, and ureteral cancer and small-intestinal cancer, may also have similar pathological characteristics. For example, the morphology of ovarian cancer arising in Lynch syndrome is typical of the endometrioid type, clear cell type or undifferentiated type [12]. However, the others have not been as well clarified.

3.6 Conclusion

The histology of colorectal cancer arising in Lynch syndrome is well known and established. Endometrial cancer in Lynch syndrome has some common histological findings with colorectal cancer. But the histology of some carcinomas in Lynch syndrome is controversial and is still not clear. Pathological findings or morphology are often useful to assess the clinicopathological background of patients and these findings may provide clues to detect patients with Lynch syndrome. Therefore, cooperation between clinicians and pathologists is needed.

Acknowledgment The authors would like to thank S Momose for providing the histological pictures (Figs. 3.1, 3.2, and 3.2) to us.

References

1. Gatalica Z, Torlakovic E. Pathology of the hereditary colorectal carcinoma. Familial Cancer. 2008;7:15–26.
2. Umar A, Boland CR, Jonathan P, et al. Revised Bethesda guidelines for hereditary nonpolyposis colorectal cancer (Lynch syndrome) and microsatellite instability. J Natl Cancer Inst. 2004;18:261–8.
3. Alexander J, Watanabe T, Wu TT, et al. Histopathological identification of colon cancer with microsatellite instability. Am J Pathol. 2001;158:527–35.
4. Jenkins MA, Hayashi S, O'shea AM, et al. Pathology features in Bethesda guidelines predict colorectal cancer microsatellite instability: a population-based study. Gastroenterology. 2007;133:48–56.
5. Bosman FT, Carneiro F, Hruban RH, et al. WHO classification of tumors of the digestive system. 4th ed. Lyon: IARC; 2010.
6. Maeda Y, Sadahiro S, Suzuki T, et al. Significance of the mucinous component in the histopathological classification of colon cancer. Surg Today. 2016;46:303–8.
7. Shen L, Toyota M, Kondo Y, et al. Integrated genetic and epigenetic analysis identifies three different subclasses of colon cancer. Proc Natl Acad Sci U S A. 2007;104(47):18654–9.
8. Nakagawa H, Nagasaka T, Cullings HM, et al. Efficient molecular screening of Lynch syndrome by specific 3′ promoter methylation of the MLH1 or BRAF mutation in colorectal cancer with high-frequency microsatellite instability. Oncl Rep. 2009;21:1577–83.
9. Kalady MF, Kravochuck SE, Heald B, et al. Defining the adenoma burden in Lynch syndrome. Dis Colon Rectum. 2015;58:388–92.
10. Mecklin JP, Aarnio M, Läärä E, et al. Development of colorectal tumors in colonoscopic surveillance in Lynch syndrome. Gastroenterology. 2007;133:1093–8.
11. Leggett B, Whitehall V. Role of the serrated pathway in colorectal cancer pathogenesis. Gastroenterology. 2010;138:2088–100.
12. Mills AM, Longacre TA. Lynch syndrome: female genital tract cancer diagnosis and screening. Surg Pathol Clin. 2016;9:201–14.
13. Garg K, Shih K, Barakat R, et al. Endometrial carcinomas in women aged 40 years and younger: tumors associated with loss of DNA mismatch repair proteins comprise a distinct clinicopathologic subset. Am J Surg Pathol. 2009;33:1869–77.
14. Tafe LJ, Garg K, Chew I, et al. Endometrial and ovarian carcinomas with undifferentiated components: clinically aggressive and frequently underrecognized neoplasms. Mod Pathol. 2010;23:781–9.
15. Saeki H, Hlaing MT, Horimot Y, et al. Usefullness of immunohistochemistry for mismatch repair protein and microsatellite instability examination in adenocarcinoma and background endometrium of sporadic endometrial cancer cases. J Obstet Gynaecol Res. 2019;45:2037–42.
16. Adar T, Rodgers LH, Shannon KM, et al. Universal screening of both endometrial and colon cancers increases the detection of Lynch syndrome. Cancer. 2018;124:3145–53.
17. Aarnio M, Salovaara R, Aaltonen LA, et al. Features of gastric cancer in hereditary nonpolyposis colorectal cancer syndrome. Int J Cancer. 1997;74:551–5.
18. Capelle LG, Grieken NCTV, Lingsma HF, et al. Risk and epidemiological time trends of gastric cancer in Lynch syndrome carriers in the Netherlands. Gastroenterology. 2010;138:487–92.
19. Saita C, Yamaguchi T, Horiguchi S, et al. Tumor development in Japanese patients with Lynch syndrome. PLoS One. 2018;13:e0195572. https://doi.org/10.1371/journal.pone.0195572.
20. Pavlidis P, Arqoub HA, Hayee BH. Gastric lesion in a patient with Lynch syndrome. Gastroenterology. 2017;153:e5–6. https://doi.org/10.1053/j.gastro.2016.12.045.
21. Giardiello FM, Allen JI, Axilbund JE, et al. Guidelines on genetic evaluation and management of Lynch syndrome: a consensus statement by the US Multi-society Task Force on colorectal cancer. Am J Gastroenterol. 2014;109:1159–79.

Immunohistochemistry for Mismatch Repair Proteins

4

Shigeki Sekine

Abstract

Immunohistochemistry for mismatch repair (MMR) proteins has been increasingly used to determine MMR status in clinical settings, including in the screening for Lynch syndrome. In addition to evaluating the MMR status, the use of immunohistochemical testing also allows the estimation of defective MMR genes, which facilitates the screening process. Immunohistochemistry can be performed on routinely processed formalin-fixed paraffin-embedded tumor specimens and the interpretation of the results is usually straightforward. However, there are several exceptional staining patterns that need to be recognized for a correct evaluation to be made. This chapter discusses the backgrounds and practical issues regarding the use of immunohistochemistry for MMR proteins in the screening process for Lynch syndrome.

Keywords

Lynch syndrome · Immunohistochemistry · Screening · Colorectal cancer Endometrial cancer

4.1 Introduction

Lynch syndrome is caused by a heterozygous germline mutation in one of the mismatch repair (MMR) genes, *MLH1*, *MSH2*, *PMS2*, or *MSH6* or the loss of *MSH2* expression due to *EPCAM* deletion [1, 2]. Patients with Lynch syndrome are associated with increased risks of several types of cancers, including colorectal,

S. Sekine (✉)
Division of Pathology and Clinical Laboratories, National Cancer Center Hospital, Tokyo, Japan
e-mail: ssekine@ncc.go.jp

N. Tomita (ed.), *Lynch Syndrome*, https://doi.org/10.1007/978-981-15-6891-6_4

endometrial, and urothelial cancers [3, 4]. Most Lynch syndrome-associated neoplasms exhibit MMR deficiency due to a somatic, in addition to a germline mutation in MMR genes. Accordingly, testing the MMR status can be used to exclude the tumors that are not associated with Lynch syndrome. Additionally, recent studies have shown a close correlation between MMR statuses and response to immune checkpoint inhibitors [5, 6]. Based on this notion, the MMR status has also been recognized as an excellent predictive biomarker to immune checkpoint inhibitors.

There are two different tests used to determine the MMR status in clinical settings: immunohistochemistry for MMR proteins and microsatellite instability (MSI) testing. Both tests can be performed on routinely processed formalin-fixed paraffin-embedded tumor specimens. Although these two tests employ totally different methodologies, their results are highly concordant with regard to the determination of the MMR status [7, 8]. Currently, immunohistochemistry for MMR proteins is generally preferred over MSI testing because immunohistochemistry can be performed in most pathology laboratories and is generally associated with shorter turnaround time. In addition, MMR protein immunohistochemistry allows the estimation of the mutated MMR genes, which facilitates the screening for Lynch syndrome.

4.2 Selection of Primary Antibodies

There are several primary antibodies available for each MMR protein. In our experience, these antibodies exhibit some variability with regard to their specificity and sensitivity. Nordic immunohistochemical Quality Control (NordiQC) website (www.nordiqc.org) is one of the excellent resources that aid in choosing appropriate MMR protein antibodies for immunohistochemistry. The website also provides information on antigen retrieval methods and staining systems.

4.3 Interpretation of Staining Results

Immunohistochemical staining of the four MMR proteins, MLH1, MSH2, PMS2, and MSH6, is used to identify MMR-deficient tumors. Cells with intact MMR function retain the expression of all four MMR proteins (Fig. 4.1), whereas the loss of any MMR proteins indicates MMR deficiency. The staining results should be reported as intact or loss of expression, rather than positive or negative, to avoid the misinterpretation of positive/negative staining results as positive/negative results for MMR deficiency [9]. Immunohistochemistry for MMR proteins allows the estimation of mutated MMR genes, in addition to the MMR statuses, with high accuracy, which is a major advantage of this method over MSI testing. However, mutations in MMR genes do not always result in the isolated loss of the respective MMR protein. Table 4.1 indicates the relationship between the defective MMR genes and the results of immunohistochemical staining. As indicated, the loss of MLH1 is accompanied by the loss of PMS2, whereas the loss of MSH2 is associated with the loss of MSH6 (Fig. 4.2). In contrast, mutations in *PMS2* and *MSH6* result in the isolated

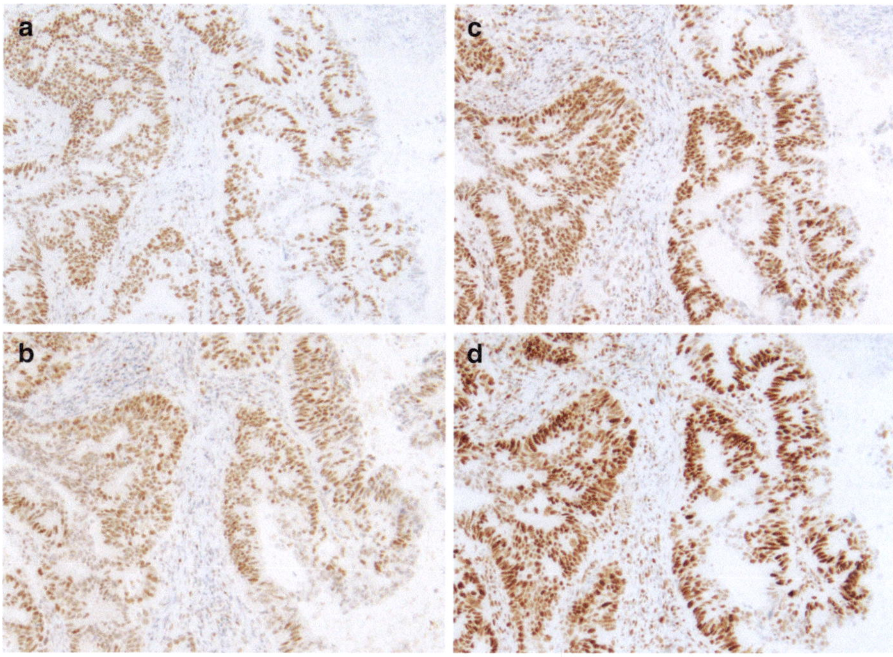

Fig. 4.1 Colon cancer with intact mismatch repair (MMR) protein expression. Four MMR proteins, MLH1 (**a**), PMS2 (**b**), MSH2 (**c**), and MSH6 (**d**), are diffusely expressed in tumor cells, indicating an intact MMR status

Table 4.1 The relationship between immunohistochemistry for mismatch repair (MMR) proteins and defective MMR genes

		Immunohistochemical expression			
		MLH1	MSH2	PMS2	MSH6
Defective MMR genes	*MLH1*	–	+	–	+
	MSH2	+	–	+	–
	PMS2	+	+	–	+
	MSH6	+	+	+	-

loss of the respective proteins they encode. These results are explained by the fact that the formation of MMR protein heterodimers is essential for their function, as well as protein stability [10].

The MMR proteins relevant to Lynch syndrome act as heterodimers. MSH2 is an essential partner of MutS complexes and can dimerize with either MSH6 or MSH3 (Fig. 4.3). Accordingly, the inactivation of MSH2 leads to the inability to form MutS complexes and the concurrent loss of MSH2 and MSH6. In contrast, MSH6 inactivation leads to the isolated loss of MSH6, since the MSH2–MSH3 heterodimer is still intact. Similarly, MLH1 is an essential component of MutL complexes and forms heterodimers with PMS2, PMS1, or MLH3. Accordingly, the inactivation

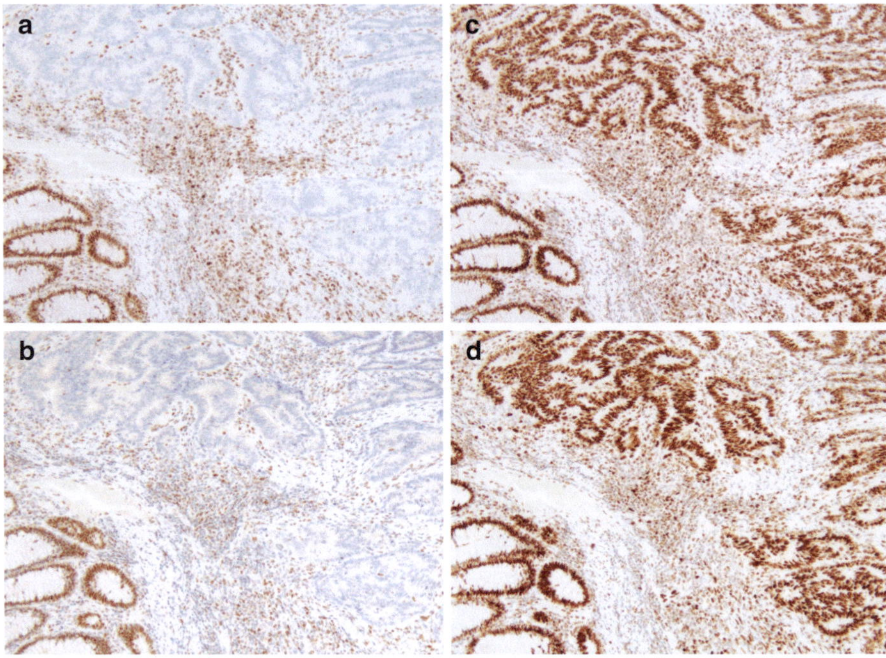

Fig. 4.2 Colon cancer in a patient with Lynch syndrome due to an *MLH1* mutation. Expression of MLH1 (**a**) and PMS2 (**b**) is lost in tumor cells, whereas the expression of MSH2 (**c**) and MSH6 (**d**) is intact, consistent with the mutation in *MLH1*. Notice that the non-neoplastic glands (lower left) and stromal cells express all the MMR proteins

of *MLH1* results in a concomitant loss of MLH1 and PMS2, but the inactivation of PMS2 leads to the isolated loss of PMS2. In each case, defects in the respective MMR genes result in specific MMR protein loss patterns, and thus, immunohistochemical testing allows us to estimate the defective MMR genes.

As in other immunohistochemical studies, a positive control is important to confirm the validity of the immunohistochemical staining for MMR proteins. Non-neoplastic proliferating cells express all four MMR proteins and serve as internal positive controls, including in samples obtained from patients with Lynch syndrome. Although the staining results typically show diffuse nuclear staining or complete loss of expression in tumors, the staining intensity may vary and some cases show significant heterogeneity, which may result from variations in fixation conditions and staining procedures. There is no consensus on the cutoff to define intact MMR protein expression. The College of American Pathologists suggests that any positive reaction in the nuclei of tumor cells should be regarded as an intact expression [9]. Some authors have suggested 5 or 10% unequivocal nuclear staining as a cutoff [11, 12].

Staining for EPCAM can be used to identify Lynch syndrome caused by *EPCAM* deletion among cases with MSH2 loss. However, the sensitivity of immunohistochemistry for EPCAM is limited because EPCAM expression is retained if a somatic mutation directly inactivates *MSH2* [13].

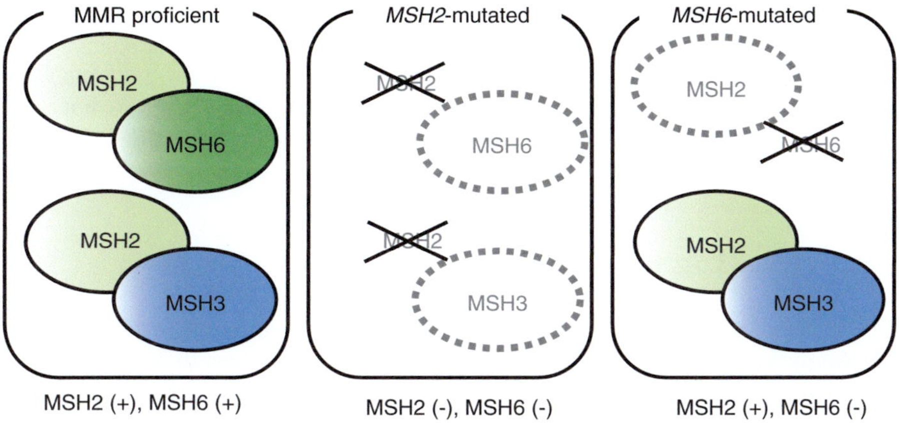

Fig. 4.3 The relationship between defects in MMR genes and protein expression in MutS complexes. MSH2 forms MutS heterodimers, which mediates mismatch recognition, with MSH6 (MutSα) or MSH3 (MutSβ). The formation of these heterodimers is critical for the stability of the proteins. Since MSH2 is an essential component of both complexes, *MSH2* mutations impair the formation of both complexes, leading to the loss of MSH6, in addition to the loss of MSH2. In contrast, mutations in *MSH6* result in the isolated loss of MSH6 because of the retention of the MSH2-MSH3 complex. Loss of MSH3 does not result in the classical MMR-deficient phenotype. A similar relationship is present between MLH1 and PMS2, which form MutL heterodimers

4.4 Exceptional Staining Results

In most cases, immunohistochemistry for MMR proteins shows either the intact expression of all four proteins or the diffuse loss of one or two proteins, as explained above. However, there are several "exceptional" staining patterns that need to be recognized for the accurate evaluation of the staining results.

4.4.1 Expression of Functionally Defective Mutant MMR Proteins

Most loss-of-function mutations in MMR genes lead to the loss of the corresponding protein products. But some mutations, particularly missense mutations, result in the expression of functionally defective proteins. This phenomenon is reportedly more common in Lynch syndrome cases with *MLH1* mutations [14]. However, these *MLH1* mutations mostly result in the isolated loss of PMS2, reflecting its dysfunction. Thus, immunohistochemical studies can effectively detect the presence of MMR deficiency in most cases with missense *MLH1* mutations.

However, it should be noted that immunohistochemical testing cannot detect any abnormalities in some cases that show the expression of functionally defective MMR proteins. If the clinical findings strongly suggest Lynch syndrome, the use of MSI testing should be considered even if the expression of all the MMR proteins is found to be intact.

4.4.2 Loss of MSH6 Associated with Neoadjuvant Chemotherapy

Colorectal cancers treated by neoadjuvant chemotherapy may exhibit significantly reduced or nucleolar MSH6 expression [15, 16]. Generally, these cases are not associated with germline *MSH6* mutations. Reanalysis of a pretreatment biopsy specimen will provide reliable results in these cases.

4.4.3 Focal Loss of MMR Proteins

MMR deficiency occurs at the early stages in the tumorigenesis of Lynch syndrome-associated colorectal cancers. Accordingly, the loss of MMR proteins is principally diffuse, and this justifies the use of biopsy specimens for the immunohistochemical analysis of MMR proteins [17, 18]. However, the focal loss of MMR proteins may be observed, in association with the diffuse loss of other MMR proteins. The most common example of this is the focal loss of MSH6 in association with the diffuse loss of MLH1 and PMS2 (Fig. 4.4). This phenomenon is attributable to the secondary mutation of *MSH6*. *MSH6* contains three mononucleotide repeats in its coding sequence (A7, C8, T7), and frameshift mutations in these repeat sequences have been observed in colorectal cancers with the focal loss of MSH6 [15, 19].

4.4.4 Abnormal Localization of MMR Proteins

Few examples of the cytoplasmic localization of MSH2 have been described, including a case with a germline *EPCAM–MSH2* fusion (Fig. 4.5) [20].

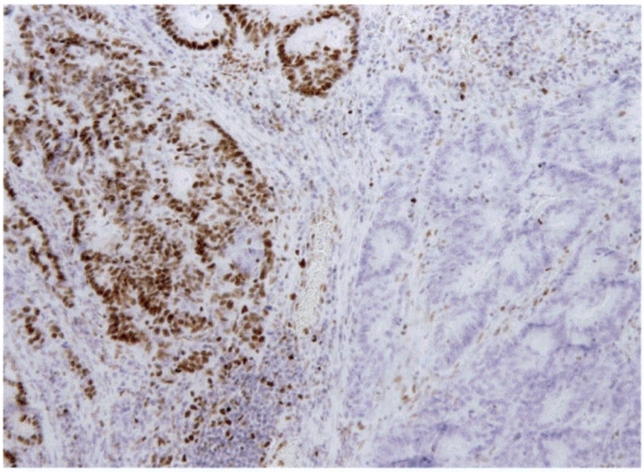

Fig. 4.4 Heterogeneous loss of MSH6 in a colon cancer. This colon cancer specimen from a Lynch syndrome patient with an *MLH1* germline mutation shows a heterogeneous loss of MSH6, in addition to the diffuse loss of MLH1 and PMS2

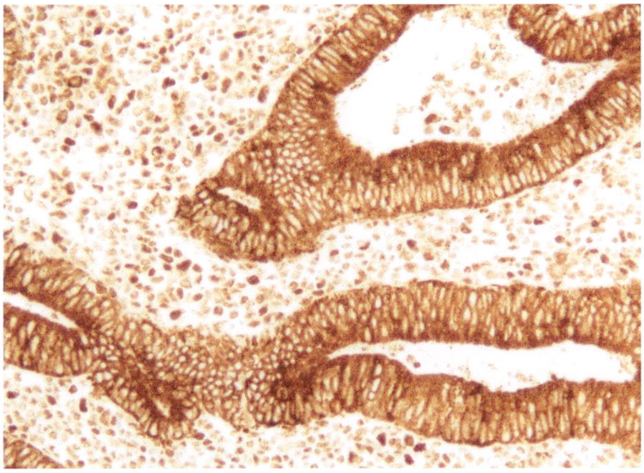

Fig. 4.5 Colon cancer exhibiting cytoplasmic MSH2 expression. A colon cancer in a patient with Lynch syndrome with a germline *EPCAM–MSH2* fusion shows MSH2 expression exclusively in the cytoplasm in tumor cells

4.4.5 Constitutional MMR Deficiency

Since patients with Lynch syndrome harbor heterozygous mutations of MMR genes, the immunohistochemical expression of MMR proteins is retained in non-neoplastic tissues [21, 22]. However, patients with constitutional MMR deficiency have homozygous MMR gene mutations, and thus, MMR protein expression is entirely lost in all cells, including non-tumoral cells. In addition to cancers commonly seen in patients with Lynch syndrome, glioblastoma, and lymphoma are frequent in patients with constitutional MMR deficiency and the age of tumor onset is usually early, often in the first decade of life.

4.4.6 False-Positive Expression of MLH1

Some studies have reported punctate nuclear MLH1 expression, in association with the loss of PMS2, in tumors with *MLH1* promoter methylation [23, 24]. A study has reported that this paradoxical MLH1 expression was seen with the use of the anti-MLH1 antibody clone M1 but not with the use of clone ES05, implying that this may be related to the use of certain anti-MLH1 antibodies [23].

4.4.7 Expression of MSH6 in MSH2-Deficient Tumors

Mutations in *MSH2* principally result in the concomitant loss of MSH2 and MSH6 expression. However, with the use of sensitive anti-MSH6 antibodies, MSH6 expression can be detectable in *MSH2*-deficient tumors (Fig. 4.6) [25]. Even in these cases, MSH6 expression is usually weaker compared with that in non-neoplastic cells.

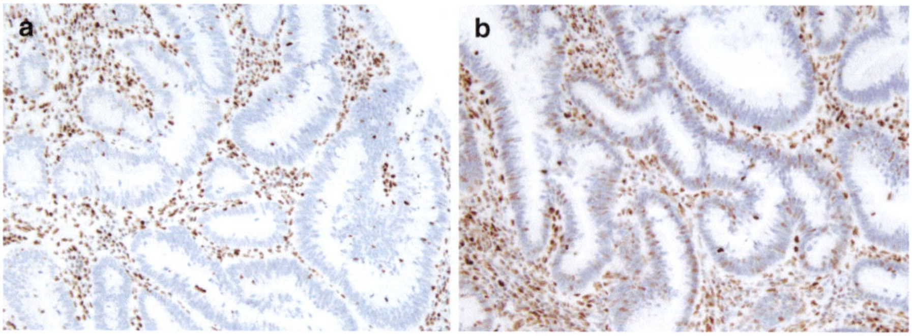

Fig. 4.6 Weak heterogeneous expression of MSH6 in a colon cancer with the loss of MSH2. Tumor cells showing a diffuse loss of MSH2 (**a**). Heterogeneous expression of MSH6 is seen but the staining intensity is considerably weaker, compared to that in non-neoplastic stromal cells (**b**). A germline *MSH2* mutation was identified in this patient

4.5 Screening Patients with Colorectal Cancers for Lynch Syndrome

There are several algorithms suggested for screening colorectal cancer patients for Lynch syndrome using immunohistochemistry. Although there are some differences among these algorithms, they all integrate the analyses for *BRAF* mutations and/or *MLH1* promoter methylation to reduce the number of cases subjected to the germline mutation analysis. After the exclusion of tumors with intact MMR protein expression by immunohistochemical testing, a significant proportion of sporadic MMR-deficient tumors can be excluded by performing these additional molecular tests.

Most sporadic MMR-deficient colorectal cancers show the loss of MLH1 expression due to *MLH1* promoter methylation, whereas tumors with *MSH2*, *PMS2*, and *MSH6* mutations are more likely to be associated with Lynch syndrome [26]. Furthermore, the *BRAF* V600E mutation has been specifically identified in sporadic cases among MLH1-deficient colorectal cancers [27, 28]. Thus, the number of patients subjected to germline mutation testing can be considerably reduced by using analyses for the *BRAF* V600E mutation and/or *MLH1* promoter methylation, in addition to immunohistochemistry.

However, it should be noted that many, but not all colorectal cancers with *MSH2*, *PMS2*, and *MSH6* mutations are associated with Lynch syndrome. Additionally, a minor subset of sporadic colorectal cancers with loss of *MLH1* lacks *MLH1* promoter methylation and instead, harbor inactivating *MLH1* mutations. These sporadic MMR-deficient colorectal cancers with somatic MMR gene mutations are called "Lynch syndrome-like tumors" [29, 30]. Since these tumors are negative for the *BRAF* V600E mutation and lack *MLH1* promoter methylation, they could not be distinguished from Lynch syndrome-associated colorectal cancers without somatic and/or germline MMR gene sequencing. Thus, while the combinatorial use of immunohistochemistry and other ancillary tests enables the efficient screening for Lynch syndrome-associated colorectal cancers, the definitive diagnosis of Lynch syndrome requires the identification of a germline mutation.

Colorectal adenomas may be used to screen for Lynch syndrome. However, a subset of adenomas, particularly, small low-grade adenomas obtained from Lynch syndrome patients retain MMR protein expression [31–33]. Thus, screening using colorectal adenoma specimens is associated with reduced sensitivity. Metastatic tumor specimens are suitable for screening for Lynch syndrome, since a high concordance between primary and metastatic tumors has been reported [34].

4.6 Screening Patients with Tumors Other than Colorectal Cancers for Lynch Syndrome

Endometrial cancer is another important and common Lynch syndrome-associated malignancy, and screening endometrial cancer patients for Lynch syndrome is appropriate [8, 35]. The major problem with screening endometrial cancers is the high prevalence of sporadic cases with MMR deficiency. Approximately 20–30% of sporadic endometrial cancers show MMR deficiency with loss of MLH1 expression [36]. Unfortunately, *BRAF* mutation testing could not be used to exclude sporadic cases in tumors other than colorectal cancer, but the analysis of *MLH1* promoter methylation is an effective way to exclude sporadic cases also in screening endometrial cancers [8]. If *MLH1* promoter methylation analysis is not available, clinicopathological findings, including the age, personal medical history, family history, and tumor morphology of the patients may be used to identify subjects with a higher risk of Lynch syndrome [37, 38]. However, screening based on clinicopathological findings would miss a portion of Lynch syndrome patients [39].

Urothelial carcinoma, particularly that in the upper urinary tract, is also a known Lynch syndrome-associated neoplasm. Previous studies have suggested that the prevalence of Lynch syndrome among cases with upper urothelial carcinomas is 1–5%, which may justify the universal screening for Lynch syndrome [40–42].

Sebaceous neoplasms of the skin are also a complication of Lynch syndrome (Fig. 4.7). Despite their limited prevalence, screening patients with sebaceous neoplasms associated with Lynch syndrome may be worth considering because of the rarity of sporadic skin sebaceous neoplasms [43].

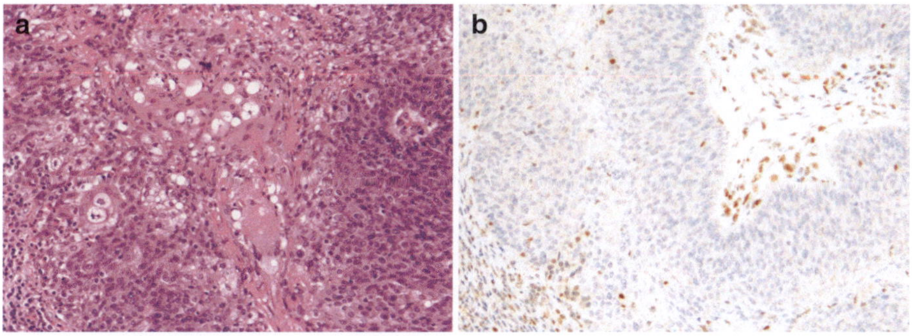

Fig. 4.7 Sebaceous carcinoma in a patient with Lynch syndrome. Sebaceous carcinoma focally exhibiting foamy cytoplasm (**a**). Tumor cells showing a diffuse loss of MSH2 (**b**)

4.7 Conclusions

Immunohistochemistry for MMR proteins, which allows the efficient identification of MMR-deficient tumors, is an important tool in screening for Lynch syndrome patients. However, the interpretation of staining results is not always straightforward because of the technical issues or unusual staining patterns. Understanding the molecular backgrounds underlying abnormal MMR protein expression and the recognition of atypical staining patterns is important for the correct evaluation of the MMR protein immunohistochemistry and the proper identification of patients at risk for Lynch syndrome.

References

1. Vasen HF. Review article: the Lynch syndrome (hereditary nonpolyposis colorectal cancer). Aliment Pharmacol Ther. 2007;26(Suppl 2):113–26.
2. Lynch HT, Snyder CL, Shaw TG, Heinen CD, Hitchins MP. Milestones of Lynch syndrome: 1895–2015. Nat Rev Cancer. 2015;15:181–94.
3. Barrow E, Hill J, Evans DG. Cancer risk in Lynch syndrome. Familial Cancer. 2013;12:229–40.
4. Bonadona V, Bonaiti B, Olschwang S, et al. Cancer risks associated with germline mutations in MLH1, MSH2, and MSH6 genes in Lynch syndrome. JAMA. 2011;305:2304–10.
5. Le DT, Uram JN, Wang H, et al. PD-1 blockade in tumors with mismatch-repair deficiency. N Engl J Med. 2015;372:2509–20.
6. Le DT, Durham JN, Smith KN, et al. Mismatch repair deficiency predicts response of solid tumors to PD-1 blockade. Science. 2017;357:409–13.
7. Shia J. Immunohistochemistry versus microsatellite instability testing for screening colorectal cancer patients at risk for hereditary nonpolyposis colorectal cancer syndrome. Part I. The utility of immunohistochemistry. J Mol Diagn. 2008;10:293–300.
8. Stelloo E, Jansen AML, Osse EM, et al. Practical guidance for mismatch repair-deficiency testing in endometrial cancer. Ann Oncol. 2017;28:96–102.
9. Bartley AN, Hamilton SR, Alsabeh R, et al. Template for reporting results of biomarker testing of specimens from patients with carcinoma of the colon and rectum. Arch Pathol Lab Med. 2014;138:166–70.
10. Boland CR, Koi M, Chang DK, Carethers JM. The biochemical basis of microsatellite instability and abnormal immunohistochemistry and clinical behavior in Lynch syndrome: from bench to bedside. Familial Cancer. 2008;7:41–52.
11. Chen W, Frankel WL. A practical guide to biomarkers for the evaluation of colorectal cancer. Mod Pathol. 2019;32(Suppl 1):1–15.
12. Pai RK, Pai RK. A practical approach to the evaluation of gastrointestinal tract carcinomas for Lynch syndrome. Am J Surg Pathol. 2016;40:e17–34.
13. Kloor M, Voigt AY, Schackert HK, et al. Analysis of EPCAM protein expression in diagnostics of Lynch syndrome. J Clin Oncol. 2011;29:223–7.
14. de Jong AE, van Puijenbroek M, Hendriks Y, et al. Microsatellite instability, immunohistochemistry, and additional PMS2 staining in suspected hereditary nonpolyposis colorectal cancer. Clin Cancer Res. 2004;10:972–80.
15. Shia J, Zhang L, Shike M, et al. Secondary mutation in a coding mononucleotide tract in MSH6 causes loss of immunoexpression of MSH6 in colorectal carcinomas with MLH1/PMS2 deficiency. Mod Pathol. 2013;26:131–8.
16. Bao F, Panarelli NC, Rennert H, Sherr DL, Yantiss RK. Neoadjuvant therapy induces loss of MSH6 expression in colorectal carcinoma. Am J Surg Pathol. 2010;34:1798–804.

17. Kumarasinghe AP, de Boer B, Bateman AC, Kumarasinghe MP. DNA mismatch repair enzyme immunohistochemistry in colorectal cancer: a comparison of biopsy and resection material. Pathology. 2010;42:414–20.
18. Shia J, Stadler Z, Weiser MR, et al. Immunohistochemical staining for DNA mismatch repair proteins in intestinal tract carcinoma: how reliable are biopsy samples? Am J Surg Pathol. 2011;35:447–54.
19. Graham RP, Kerr SE, Butz ML, et al. Heterogenous MSH6 loss is a result of microsatellite instability within MSH6 and occurs in sporadic and hereditary colorectal and endometrial carcinomas. Am J Surg Pathol. 2015;39:1370–6.
20. Sekine S, Ogawa R, Saito S, et al. Cytoplasmic MSH2 immunoreactivity in a patient with Lynch syndrome with an EPCAM-MSH2 fusion. Histopathology. 2017;70:664–9.
21. Wimmer K, Kratz CP, Vasen HF, et al. Diagnostic criteria for constitutional mismatch repair deficiency syndrome: suggestions of the European consortium 'care for CMMRD' (C4CMMRD). J Med Genet. 2014;51:355–65.
22. Vasen HF, Ghorbanoghli Z, Bourdeaut F, et al. Guidelines for surveillance of individuals with constitutional mismatch repair-deficiency proposed by the European Consortium "Care for CMMR-D" (C4CMMR-D). J Med Genet. 2014;51:283–93.
23. Niu BT, Hammond RFL, Leen SLS, et al. Artefactual punctate MLH1 staining can lead to erroneous reporting of isolated PMS2 loss. Histopathology. 2018;73:703–5.
24. Loughrey MB, Dunne PD, Coleman HG, McQuaid S, James JA. Punctate MLH1 mismatch repair immunostaining in colorectal cancer. Histopathology. 2018;74(5):795–7.
25. Pearlman R, Markow M, Knight D, et al. Two-stain immunohistochemical screening for Lynch syndrome in colorectal cancer may fail to detect mismatch repair deficiency. Mod Pathol. 2018;31:1891–900.
26. Kane MF, Loda M, Gaida GM, et al. Methylation of the hMLH1 promoter correlates with lack of expression of hMLH1 in sporadic colon tumors and mismatch repair-defective human tumor cell lines. Cancer Res. 1997;57:808–11.
27. Parsons MT, Buchanan DD, Thompson B, Young JP, Spurdle AB. Correlation of tumour BRAF mutations and MLH1 methylation with germline mismatch repair (MMR) gene mutation status: a literature review assessing utility of tumour features for MMR variant classification. J Med Genet. 2012;49:151–7.
28. Adar T, Rodgers LH, Shannon KM, et al. A tailored approach to BRAF and MLH1 methylation testing in a universal screening program for Lynch syndrome. Mod Pathol. 2017;30:440–7.
29. Mensenkamp AR, Vogelaar IP, van Zelst-Stams WA, et al. Somatic mutations in MLH1 and MSH2 are a frequent cause of mismatch-repair deficiency in Lynch syndrome-like tumors. Gastroenterology. 2014;146:643–6.e8.
30. Rodriguez-Soler M, Perez-Carbonell L, Guarinos C, et al. Risk of cancer in cases of suspected lynch syndrome without germline mutation. Gastroenterology. 2013;144:926–32.e1; quiz e13-4.
31. De Jong AE, Morreau H, Van Puijenbroek M, et al. The role of mismatch repair gene defects in the development of adenomas in patients with HNPCC. Gastroenterology. 2004;126:42–8.
32. Sekine S, Mori T, Ogawa R, et al. Mismatch repair deficiency commonly precedes adenoma formation in Lynch syndrome-associated colorectal tumorigenesis. Mod Pathol. 2017;30:1144–51.
33. Yurgelun MB, Goel A, Hornick JL, et al. Microsatellite instability and DNA mismatch repair protein deficiency in Lynch syndrome colorectal polyps. Cancer Prev Res (Phila). 2012;5:574–82.
34. Haraldsdottir S, Roth R, Pearlman R, et al. Mismatch repair deficiency concordance between primary colorectal cancer and corresponding metastasis. Familial Cancer. 2016;15:253–60.
35. Hampel H, Frankel W, Panescu J, et al. Screening for Lynch syndrome (hereditary nonpolyposis colorectal cancer) among endometrial cancer patients. Cancer Res. 2006;66:7810–7.
36. Cancer Genome Atlas Research N, Kandoth C, Schultz N, et al. Integrated genomic characterization of endometrial carcinoma. Nature. 2013;497:67–73.

37. Rabban JT, Calkins SM, Karnezis AN, et al. Association of tumor morphology with mismatch-repair protein status in older endometrial cancer patients: implications for universal versus selective screening strategies for Lynch syndrome. Am J Surg Pathol. 2014;38:793–800.
38. Moline J, Mahdi H, Yang B, et al. Implementation of tumor testing for lynch syndrome in endometrial cancers at a large academic medical center. Gynecol Oncol. 2013;130:121–6.
39. Mills AM, Liou S, Ford JM, et al. Lynch syndrome screening should be considered for all patients with newly diagnosed endometrial cancer. Am J Surg Pathol. 2014;38:1501–9.
40. Ju JY, Mills AM, Mahadevan MS, et al. Universal Lynch syndrome screening should be performed in all upper tract urothelial carcinomas. Am J Surg Pathol. 2018;42:1549–55.
41. Harper HL, McKenney JK, Heald B, et al. Upper tract urothelial carcinomas: frequency of association with mismatch repair protein loss and lynch syndrome. Mod Pathol. 2017;30:146–56.
42. Metcalfe MJ, Petros FG, Rao P, et al. Universal point of care testing for Lynch syndrome in patients with upper tract urothelial carcinoma. J Urol. 2018;199:60–5.
43. Everett JN, Raymond VM, Dandapani M, et al. Screening for germline mismatch repair mutations following diagnosis of sebaceous neoplasm. JAMA Dermatol. 2014;150:1315–21.

Genetic Analysis for Lynch Syndrome 5

Izumi Miyabe, Keisuke Tanaka, and Kiwamu Akagi

Abstract

Genetic testing for Lynch syndrome has become increasingly important in cancer clinic, since tissue-agnostic immune checkpoint inhibitor therapy for mismatch repair deficient tumor has been approved. However, extensive effort are needed to identify pathogenic variants in LS causative genes (*MLH1*, *MSH2*, *MSH6*, *PMS2*, *EPCAM*). Therefore, efficient and time-saving method is indispensable for clinical practice. Multigene panel testing using molecular barcode and next generation sequencer (NGS) makes it possible to detect single nucleotide variants (SNVs), small indels, and copy number variations (CNVs) in the same assay. Although it is still difficult to detect some complex variants such as large insertion, inversion, complex rearrangement, and so on, these technologies will give more chances to diagnose with Lynch syndrome.

Keywords

Mismatch repair gene · *MLH1* · *MSH2* · *MSH6* · *PMS2* · *EPCAM* · Sanger sequence · Multiplex Ligation-dependent Probe Amplification (MLPA) · Next generation sequencing (NGS) · Multigene panel testing

I. Miyabe · K. Tanaka · K. Akagi (✉)
Department of Molecular Diagnosis and Cancer Prevention, Saitama Cancer Center, Saitama, Japan
e-mail: akagi@cancer-c.pref.saitama.jp

N. Tomita (ed.), *Lynch Syndrome*, https://doi.org/10.1007/978-981-15-6891-6_5

5.1 Causative Genes for Lynch Syndrome

Lynch syndrome (LS) is caused by germline pathogenic variants in the mismatch repair (MMR) genes [1]. The MMR pathway corrects single base–base or insertion/deletion (indel) mismatches resulted from misincorporation by DNA polymerases during DNA replication. Since LS is an autosomal dominant disease, a heterozygous pathogenic variant in one of four MMR genes (*MLH1*, *MSH2*, *MSH6*, *PMS2*) can cause LS. Germline deletions of the transcription terminator of *EPCAM*, which is not involved in the MMR pathway, can also cause LS through repression of expression of the adjacent gene, *MSH2* [2]. In addition to alteration of genomic DNA sequence, constitutional inactivation of *MLH1* by cytosine methylation in its promoter has been reported as a cause of LS, although it is not always inheritable [3, 4].

The MMR pathway is one of the major DNA repair mechanisms which is conserved from prokaryotes to higher eukaryotes. MutS and MutL play a central role in the MMR pathway both in prokaryotes and eukaryotes. While prokaryotic MutS and MutL function as homodimers, eukaryotes have multiple homologs of these proteins and they form heterodimers. The major MutS heterodimer in eukaryotes is MutS α comprising MSH2 (MutS homolog 2) and MSH6, (MutS homolog), which recognizes and binds a mismatch in DNA. ATP and its binding to a mismatch induce a conformational change, which allows its interaction with the major MutL heterodimer, MutL α, comprising MLH1 (MutL Homolog 1) and PMS2 (homolog of yeast PMS1). Subsequently, MutL α is activated and incises the newly synthesized strand and the DNA ends are used to remove the replication error [5, 6].

Inactivation of the MMR pathway results in an elevated rate of spontaneous mutation especially indels at homopolymeric runs, which is referred to as microsatellite instability (MSI). MSI is a distinctive feature of cancers caused by LS. Germline biallelic inactivation of one of four MMR genes causes a disease called Constitutional Mismatch Repair Deficiency syndrome (CMMRD), also known as Mismatch Repair Cancer Syndrome (MMRCS) (OMIM #276300). CMMRD is a rare childhood cancer predisposition syndrome [7]. The spectrum of cancers observed in patients with CMMRD is apparently different from that found in LS. Brain tumors are the most common, followed by gastrointestinal and hematological malignancies.

5.1.1 *MLH1*

MLH1 is located on chromosome 3 at 3p22.2, ~57 kb in length. It is composed of 19 exons encoding a protein of 756 amino acids. MLH1 protein contains an ATPase domain and protein-protein interaction domains (Fig. 5.1a). MLH1 heterodimerizes with the product of *PMS2* to form MutL α. MutL α functions as a nuclease in an ATP dependent manner.

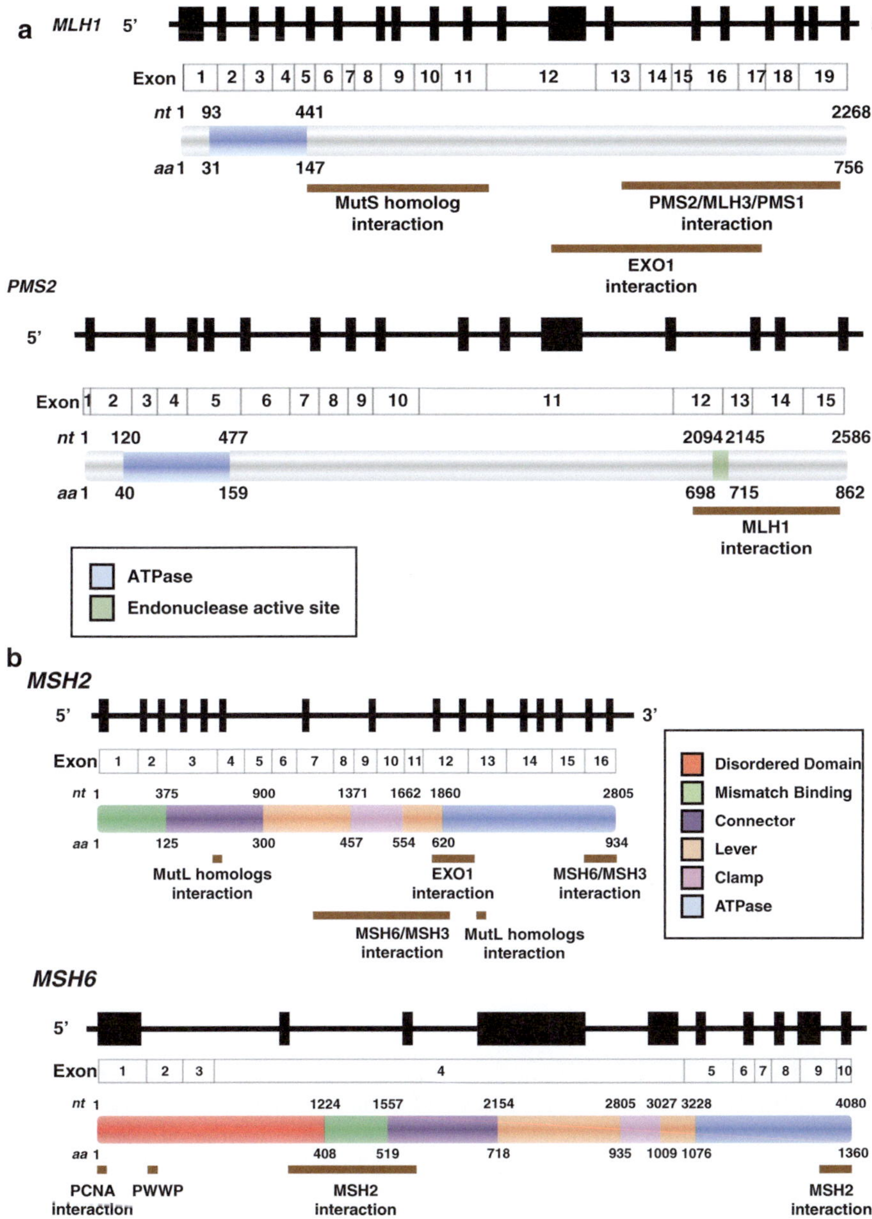

Fig. 5.1 Schematic representation of the MMR genes and proteins. (**a**) Subunits of MutL α. Upper and lower schematics show MLH1 and PMS2, respectively. (**b**) Subunits of MutS α. Upper and lower schematics show MSH2 and MSH6, respectively. Top shows exon–intron structure of the gene. Rod shows each protein with functional and interaction domains. Corresponding exons are shown above the rod. (**c**) Pseudogenes of *PMS2*. Positions of *PMS2* and *PMS2CL* genes on the chromosome 7, and homology between *PMS2* and pseudogenes are shown. Tel and Cen represent telomere and centromere, respectively

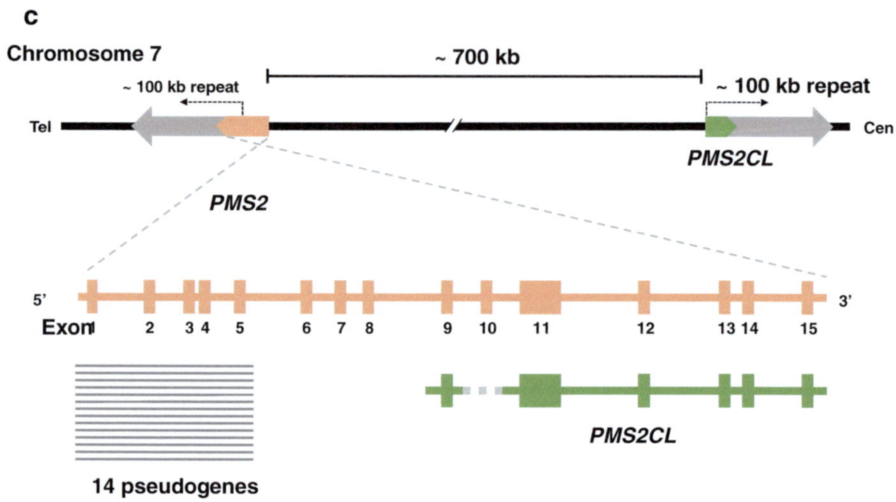

Fig. 5.1 (continued)

5.1.2 *MSH2*

MSH2 is located on chromosome 2 between 2p21 and 2p16. It is ~80 kb in length with 16 exons encoding a protein of 934 amino acids. MSH2 contains DNA binding domain, ATPase domain, and protein-protein interaction domains. It binds MSH6 to form MutS α. MSH2 and MSH6 are structurally divided into five domains. (1) the DNA mismatch binding domain, (2) Connector between the mismatch binding domain and lever, (3) Lever is interrupted by (4) Clamp, which allows for nonspecific DNA binding. The lever and clamp are required for the conformational change of the heterodimer. (5) ATPase domain (Fig. 5.1b).

5.1.3 *MSH6*

MSH6 is located at 2p16.3, ~300 kb downstream of *MSH2*. It is ~24 kb in length and composed of 10 exons encoding a protein of 1360 amino acids. In addition to five domains seen in MutS homologs, MSH6 has a unique disordered domain at its N-terminus. The N-terminal domain contains a PCNA (proliferating cell nuclear antigen) binding motif, PWWP sequences which provide nonspecific DNA-protein binding, and multiple phosphorylation sites (Fig. 5.1b).

5.1.4 *PMS2*

PMS2 is located at 7p22 and ~36 kb in length. Fifteen exons encode a protein of 862 amino acids. PMS2 heterodimerize with MLH1. The C-terminal domain of PMS2 binds to MLH1 and contains the endonuclease active site which is responsible for the incision of the nascent strand.

Genetic analysis of *PMS2* is difficult because of the presence of numerous pseudogenes. Fifteen pseudogenes have been identified and all of them are located on chromosome 7. Fourteen pseudogenes bear a similarity to some or all of exon 1–5 of *PMS2*, whereas the *PMS2CL* (*PMS2* C-terminal Like pseudogene) is highly homologous with exon 9 and 11–15 (Fig. 5.1c) [8, 9]. *PMS2CL* presents in a large inverted repeat (~100 kb) and sequence transfer between *PMS2CL* and *PMS2* has been reported [10, 11]. This nature makes variant analysis of *PMS2* difficult and inaccurate. Therefore, 3′ terminus of *PMS2* needs to be analyzed separately (see below).

5.1.5 *EPCAM*

EPCAM is located at 2p21, ~16 kb upstream of *MSH2*. It is composed of 9 exons encoding a protein of 862 amino acids. EPCAM itself is not involved in the MMR pathway. However, when the transcription terminator of *EPCAM* is deleted, the transcription continues to *MSH2*. This results in the silencing of *MSH2* by promoter methylation.

5.1.6 Other MMR Genes

Although the vast majority of mismatches are repaired by MutS α and MutL α, other MutS and MutL heterodimers are known to participate in the MMR pathway. For example, the MutS β (MSH2-MSH3 heterodimer) repairs large indels as well as one or two base indel mismatches. With regard to MutL, MLH1 can heterodimerize with PMS1 or MLH3 as well as PMS2. Correlation between these alternative MMR genes and cancer predisposition is still uncertain although several reports have been published [12, 13].

5.2 Pathogenic Variants in Genes Causing LS

5.2.1 Contribution of Causative Genes to LS

As of September 2018, ~3300 unique variants of the MMR genes have been deposited into International Society for Gastrointestinal Hereditary Tumors (InSiGHT) locus-specific database. Variants in *MLH1*, *MSH2*, *MSH6*, and *PMS2* account for 40.3, 34.1, 18.2, and 7.4%, respectively (Fig. 5.2a). Since quite a few variants of *EPCAM* are listed in this database and they are not classified, *EPCAM* variants are not included in the chart.

The clinical classification of variants in disease-related genes significantly influence clinical actions to be taken for patients and their relatives. InSiGHT has

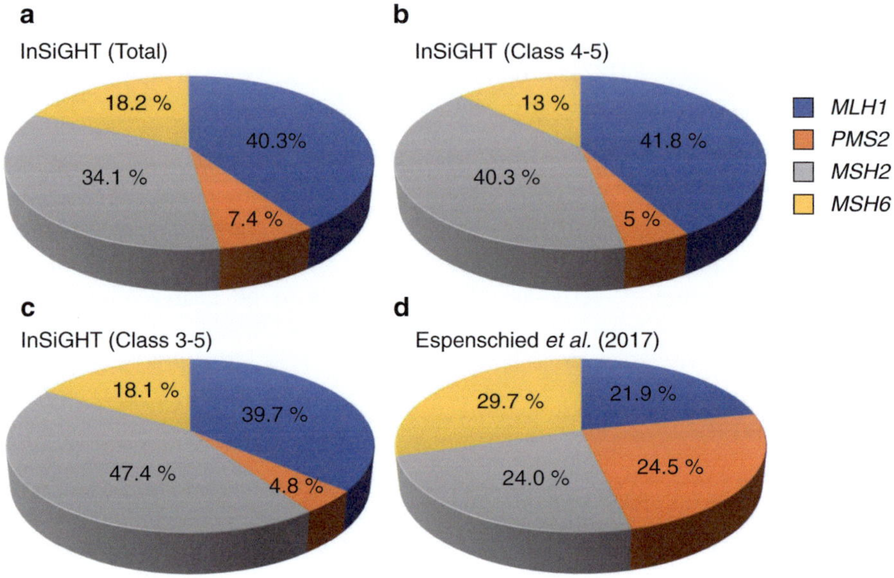

Fig. 5.2 Distribution of variants in the MMR genes. Data from (**a**) InSiGHT Class 1–5 (**b**) InSiGHT Class 4–5 (**c**) InSiGHT Class 3–5 (**d**) Espenschied et al. [14] are shown. *EPCAM* deletions are excluded

developed criteria for classifying pathogenicity of variants in the MMR genes. Out of ~3300 variants, ~1240 and ~200 are classified as "Class 5" (Pathogenic) and "Class 4" (Likely pathogenic), respectively. Focused on "Class4/Class 5" (Likely pathogenic/Pathogenic) variants, the proportion of *MLH1* is approximately equal to that of *MSH2* and higher than that of *MSH6*. The proportion of *PMS2* is the smallest among four MMR genes (Fig. 5.2b). When it is extended to variants that potentially cause the disease, i.e., from Class 3 to 5, the pattern is still similar to that of total variants (Fig. 5.2c). Therefore, pathogenic variants in *MLH1* or *MSH2* have been thought to be the main cause of LS.

However, the landscape of LS causative genes is changing because of the advance in genetic testing with next generation sequencing (NGS). Recent studies employing multigene panel testing show totally different profile of LS [14, 15]. The multigene panel testing allows clinicians to test multiple genes simultaneously in a cost-effective manner (see below). According to these studies, the frequency of variants in four MMR genes is approximately equal (Fig. 5.2d). Higher frequency of *MSH6* or *PMS2* variants is at least partly due to the difference in the selection of individuals who undergo a genetic testing for the MMR genes. Traditionally, genetic testing for LS was recommended to patients based on their personal or family history of cancer. Genetic testing for LS was first applied to families that met Amsterdam I criteria, followed by Amsterdam II criteria [16, 17]. These strict screening for patients to undergo genetic testing might have caused a bias in favor of *MLH1* and *MSH2*. Once it was revealed that MSI was a hallmark of LS cancer, new clinical criteria for LS, Bethesda Guideline, was developed [18, 19]. More recently, universal screening for LS has been implemented in a number of institutes using MSI testing and immunohistochemistry (IHC). Although MSI and IHC are effective as screening tools, some LS patients may still be missed. In addition, their sensitivity is relatively low for cancers caused by inactivation of *MSH6* and *PMS2*. Using multigene panel testing, Espenschied et al. showed 27.3% of patients in their cohort did not meet any of current criteria for LS testing and 15.2% of MSI and/or IHC results for *MSH6* or *PMS2* carriers were discordant. These patients might have been missed without a multigene panel testing. In addition, they found that *MSH6* and *PMS2* carriers were more frequent than *MLH1* and *MSH2* carriers among patients with breast cancer. This is consistent with a recent study reported by Robert et al. [19]. Although MutL α and MutS α repair the majority of mismatches in DNA, phenotypes are apparently different between subunits. For example, LS families of *PMS2* carriers have lower penetrance than that of *MLH1* carriers [20, 21]. Further genetic testing with multigene panel will reveal more LS patients who may be missed by traditional criteria based testing and facilitate understanding of the etiology of LS.

5.3 Distributions of the Types of Germline Variants in MMR Genes

Figure 5.3 shows distributions of variants listed in InSiGHT database by the types of mutations. After excluding Class 1/Class 2 (Benign/Likely benign) variants that are suggested not to cause LS, nonsense and frameshift variants are the most frequent for all MMR genes. Although missense variants, which result in amino acid substitutions, account for significant proportion (25–42%), the share of these variants is significantly decreased when Class 3 (Uncertain significance) is removed. InSiGHT Variant Interpretation Committee (VIC) is trying to interpret the pathogenicity of each variant, based on patient/family history and/or various functional assays. However, the significant number of missense variants remain Class 3. Approximately 70% of Class 3 variants are missense for all MMR genes. Class 3 variants, also referred to as Variants with Uncertain Significance (VUS), put burden on patients, clinicians, and genetic counselors. Further effort is required to understand the correlation between variants and diseases.

In addition to base substitutions and small indels, the share of large genomic rearrangements (LGRs) is also significant especially in Class 4–5 panels (Fig. 5.3 right panels). Repetitive Alu sequence-mediated ectopic recombination is suggested to promote LGRs. It has been reported that rearrangements suggested to be mediated by Alu repeats are seen in both *MLH1* and *MSH2* [22]. The fact that the proportion of this kind of LGRs is higher for *MSH2* than for *MLH1* may explain the higher frequency of LGRs in *MSH2*. LGRs are also seen in *PMS2* at high frequency although not many pathogenic variants are listed in the database for *PMS2*. It may at least partly be explained by aberrant recombination between *PMS2* and *PMS2CL* since more than half of LGRs are observed in regions that overlap with

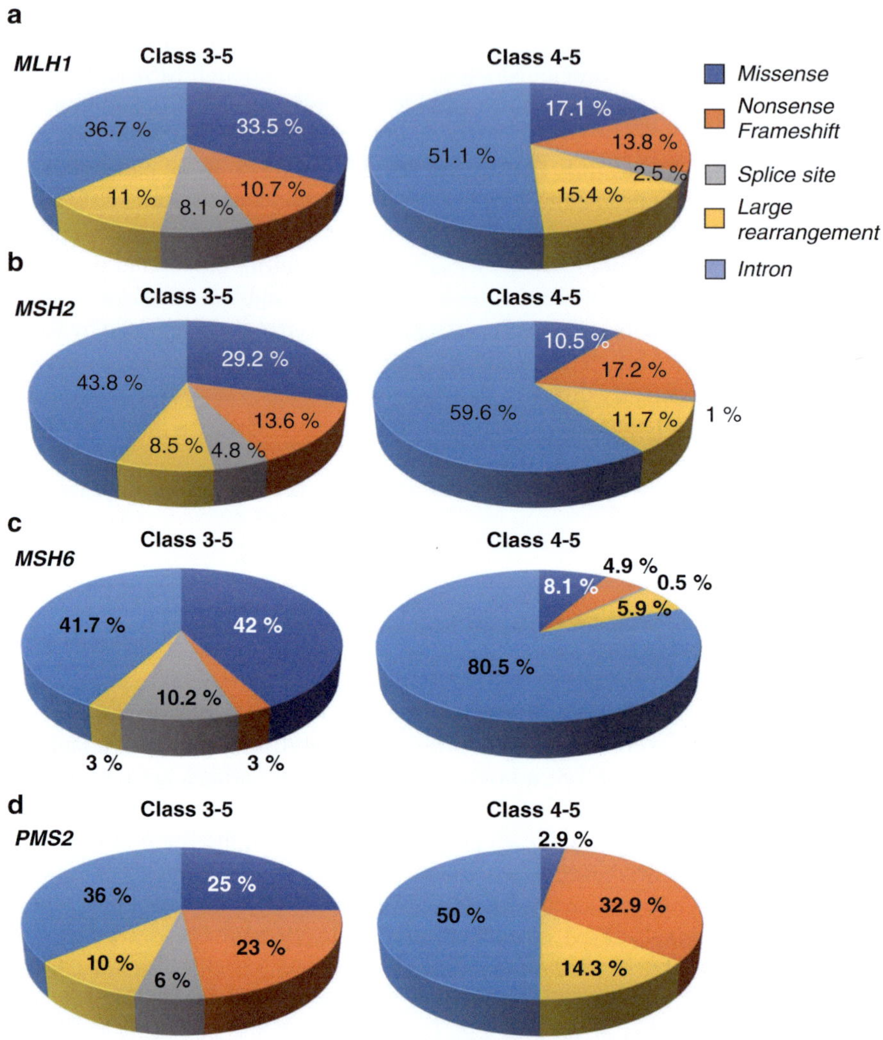

Fig. 5.3 Distribution of types of variants in each MMR gene. (**a**) *MLH1*, (**b**) *MSH2*, (**c**) *MSH6*, (**d**) *PMS2*. Left chart shows distribution of Class 3–5 variants. Right shows that of Class 4–5. Minor variants such as variants in start codon are excluded

PMS2CL. However, exact break points of LGR have not been identified in most cases because they are detected as copy number variants. Characterization of these LGR may facilitate understanding the importance of LGR in the etiology of LS and the development of genetic testing to detect LGR.

Variants within splice sites are also one of the significant causes of LS. These variants induce splicing errors such as deletion of an exon and indels by using cryptic splice sites, resulting in large deletions, frameshift, and in-frame indels at mRNA level. In addition to variants in splicing sites, some of variants inside exon (or intron outside splice sites) cause splicing error by disrupting splice sites or creating alternative splice sites [23]. Therefore, even silent variants can affect splicing and cause LS. Careful characterization is required for the accurate interpretation of pathogenicity of variants.

5.4 Genetic Testing for Lynch Syndrome

The definitive diagnosis of LS is decided by germline genetic testing. However, as described above, various sequence aberrations occur in MMR genes, such as substitution, small indels, large indels, splicing abnormality, and complex rearrangement, several methods are sometimes required to detect variant. The recent advance of technologies on NGS made it possible to detect both single nucleotide variants (SNVs), small indels, and copy number variations in the same assay.

5.4.1 Sanger Sequencing

Sanger sequencing, also known as dideoxy sequencing method, is the traditional method to determine the sequence of DNA. Many clinical laboratories and research institutes have employed this method before the advent of NGS. The difference between Sanger sequence and NGS is the volume of sequencing at a single run. Sanger sequencing is fast and cost effective when the target number is small. When sequencing small region(s) of a few samples, Sanger sequence is useful, however, genes are composed of a number of exons. When a whole gene composed of a lot of exons or included large exon is sequenced, all of exons or coding regions must be amplified and sequenced separately (Fig. 5.1a). For example, *MLH1* has 19 exons (Fig. 5.4a). To read all coding sequences of *MLH1* by Sanger sequencing, 18 pairs of primer are necessary (Exon7 and exon8 are closely located and can be analyzed together). More than 60 PCR reactions are required to sequence all exons of four MMR genes [24]. Since it is very time-consuming and labor-intensive way for clinical laboratories, it is practically impossible to conduct genetic testing for many patients. This is one of the reasons why genetic testing has been limited to patients who meet clinical criteria based on patient and family history.

5.4.2 MLPA (Multiplex Ligation-Dependent Probe Amplification)

MLPA is a PCR-based method to detect CNVs. As described above, a significant proportion of LS causative variants is that of LGRs including deletions and duplications of whole exon(s). In order to detect such genomic abnormality by MLPA, two probes that are complementary to the target region are designed. Probes hybridize

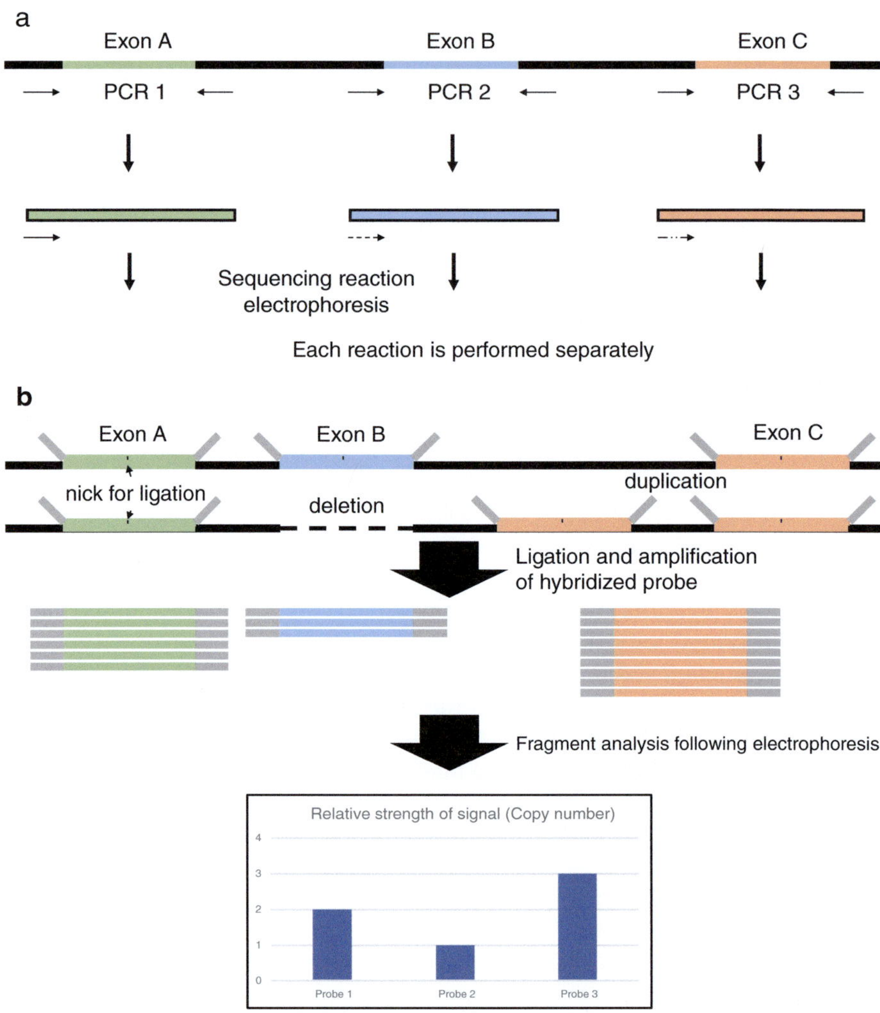

Fig. 5.4 Schematic representation of Sanger sequencing and MLPA. (**a**) Sanger sequencing. Each PCR reaction contains a single pair of primers and each PCR product is sequenced individually. (**b**) MLPA. Probes complementary to the targets of interest are hybridized with genomic DNA. The top allele represents a normal allele. In the bottom allele, Exon A presents normally, Exon B is deleted, and Exon C is tandemly duplicated. After ligation of paired probes, probes are amplified with universal primers, followed by quantification of PCR products. The graph shows an expected result

to adjacent sequences forming ligatable nick (Fig. 5.4b). After ligation, hybridized probes are amplified by PCR with fluorescent-labeled universal primers. PCR products are separated through electrophoresis according to the length. Relative strength of fluorescent signal indicates the copy number of the target region. MLPA has a weak point that false negative or positive is shown when sequence variant(s) are located in the region the probe is designed [22]. Sequence variants in the target region cause an underestimation of the copy number since they reduce the efficiency of hybridization and result in weaker fluorescent signal. It may lead to wrong conclusions. For example, a weaker signal apparently looks like a deletion of the target region when it happens in a region with normal copy number. On the other hand, if it happens in a duplicated region, the duplication may be missed. MLPA should be combined with the sequencing.

5.4.3 Next Generation Sequencing (NGS)

NGS is becoming more popular method to identify the variants of the genes causing LS as well as the other hereditary disease [25]. NGS technology enabled us to read a large number of genes simultaneously (Fig. 5.5a). The variants NGS technology can detect are not limited to substitution, small deletion, and insertion. Even large deletion and duplication spanning the multiple exons can be detected with NGS by comparing the coverage (The number of reads that cover the target region) (Fig. 5.5b). The cost to introduce the NGS technology to a

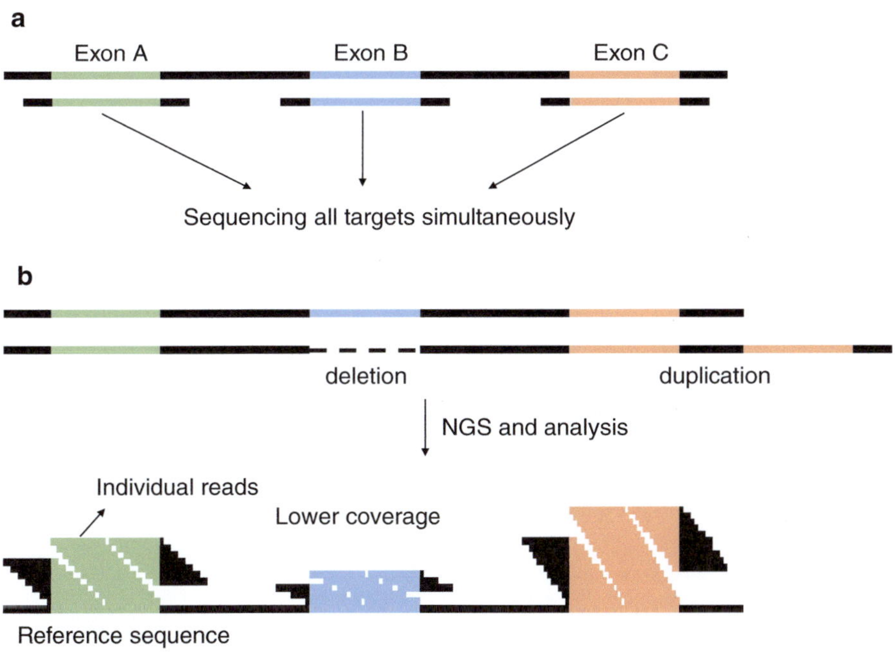

Fig. 5.5 Amplicon sequencing and quantification of the copy number by NGS. (**a**) Regions of interest are amplified by multiplex (or one by one) PCR. All of products are processed and sequenced in a single tube. (**b**) Alleles are the same as Fig. 5.4b. Bottom cartoon shows a pattern of mapping. The number of reads mapped on the deleted or duplicated exon is reduced or increased, respectively

clinical laboratory has gotten much lower compared to that of the time next generation sequencer had appeared first [26]. Thus, NGS is superseding the traditional method as the standard method to identify the variants of the genes. In following sections, the application of NGS technology for the genetic testing of LS is described.

5.4.4 Multigene Panel Testing of LS Causative Genes

The causative genes of LS are *MLH1*, *MSH2*, *MSH6*, *PMS2*, and *EPCAM* as described above. The development of "target enrichment method" made clinical laboratories familiar with NGS technology. The target enrichment method selectively isolates or amplifies target regions from genomic DNA. Whole Exome Sequencing (WES) is representative of the target enrichment method. Exons account for only about 1% of human genome. WES enriches all of exons (~180,000 in human) prior to NGS analysis. It is also possible to enrich specific subset of genes. This is often referred to as multigene panel testing. Multigene panel testing is ideal for identifying sequence variants that are associated with diseases. In case of LS, four MMR genes are primary targets to be enriched. However, phenotypes of LS overlap to other hereditary cancer syndromes, it is not efficient to confine five causative genes for genetic diagnosis. Therefore, in many clinical laboratories, multiple genes associated with hereditary gastrointestinal cancer are analyzed in addition to MMR genes and *EPCAM* as multigene panel testing (Table 5.1). The National Comprehensive Cancer Network (NCCN) guidelines list frequently chosen genes in the multigene panel for hereditary colorectal cancer such as *MLH1*, *MSH2*, *MSH6*, *PMS2*, *EPCAM*, *APC*, *MUTYH*, *POLE*, *POLD1*, and *TP53*.

Many of the panels for hereditary colorectal cancer in the clinical laboratories include all of the listed genes.

Table 5.1 Hereditary colorectal cancer syndrome and causative genes

Genes	Associated disease
MLH1	Lynch syndrome
MSH2	
MSH6	
PMS2	
EPCAM	
APC	Familial adenomatous polyposis
BMPR1A	Juvenile polyposis syndrome
MUTYH	MUTYH-associated polyposis
POLE	Polymerase proofreading-associated polyposis
POLD1	
TP53	Li-Fraumeni syndrome

5.4.5 Capture Hybridization-Based and Amplicon-Based Method

There are two methods for target enrichment, capture hybridization-based and amplicon-based method [27] (Fig. 5.6). The capture hybridization method enriches the regions of interest with hundreds bases of the hybridization probes complementary with target sequences. Longer probes than of MLPA prevent nonspecific hybridization and a fall of the hybridization efficiency by the polymorphism. However, capture hybridization-based method is less cost effective and its procedure to prepare samples is more complicated compared with the amplicon-based method. In addition, a larger amount of input DNA is required to assure adequate coverage for analysis. This causes a problem when the amount of the sample is limited. Amplicon-based method enriches the regions of interest by multiplex PCR (Fig. 5.6). The process of amplicon-based method is less complicated and the amount of input DNA can be lower. However, this method requires many cycles of PCR, so that frequency of polymerase error (The alterations not existing in the original DNA sequence is given rise) is higher and PCR bias (all targets are not amplified equally) is stronger. Thus, sequencing too many targets with amplicon-based method is not favorable. Typically, less than 50 genes (1500 targets) are

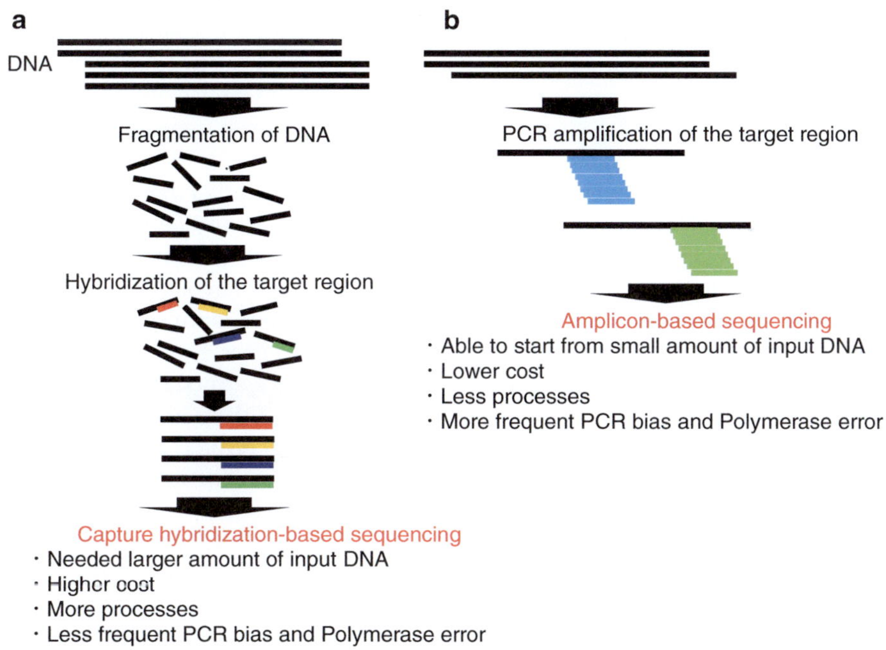

Fig. 5.6 Capture hybridization- and amplicon-based method. (**a**) Capture method. Randomly fragmented genomic DNA is hybridized with probes to enrich the regions of interest. Enriched fragments are processed to be sequenced. (**b**) Target regions are amplified by a multiplex PCR, followed by sample preparation for sequencing

sequenced by this method. Recently, modified amplicon methods have been developed and the number of targets is increasing. At present, these methods are preferred [28, 29].

5.4.6 Detection of CNVs by NGS

NGS determines the sequence of every single molecule. Millions of DNA molecules are sequenced in a single run and obtained sequences (also called "Reads") are mapped on a reference genome to analyze the sequencing result. Copy number of the target can be estimated by counting the number of reads mapped within the target locus (Actually normalization is required) (Fig. 5.5b). The capture method has an advantage over the amplicon method in this case. Although both methods require PCR amplification of DNA fragments to prepare a library, the number of cycles required for library preparation is fewer, and single primer set is used for the capture method. Therefore, the capture method causes less PCR bias. In addition, the capture method initiates from the random fragmentation of genomic DNA. Most, if not all, of fragments have unique ends because it is unlikely that independent DNA molecules are fragmented at exactly the same position at both ends. Thus, reads carrying identical ends are presumed to be derived from the same molecule. The number of reads can be normalized by removing redundant reads so that the copy number is estimated more accurately.

On the other hand, the amplicon method creates identical fragments for each target. It is impossible to remove redundant reads in the same way despite the fact that PCR bias is bigger. Therefore, it is not favorable to estimate copy number by the amplicon method. To overcome this problem, random short sequence referred to as molecular barcode is added to the end(s) of amplicon at an early point of the procedure [30]. Ten nucleotides molecular barcode can label about one million molecules. If multiple PCR products have the same barcode, they presumably originate from the same template. Once molecules with the same barcode are identified, redundant reads can be removed as shown in Fig. 5.7. Thus, normalizing the read counts by molecular barcode enables to estimate copy number.

Molecular barcode can also be used to remove sequence errors. DNA fragments with the same barcode should have identical sequences. If there is difference, it is supposed to be derived from sequencing error. Sequencing error(s) can be removed by "majority rule." Molecular barcode is applicable to the capture method as well as the amplicon method although the effect may be less dramatic.

In summary, NGS can detect SNVs, small indels, and CNVs suggestive of LGRs at the same time. However, NGS is not perfect at least for the time being. For example, the copy number estimated by NGS fluctuates depending on loci or experimental conditions. It is recommended to double-check by another method such as MLPA or quantitative PCR.

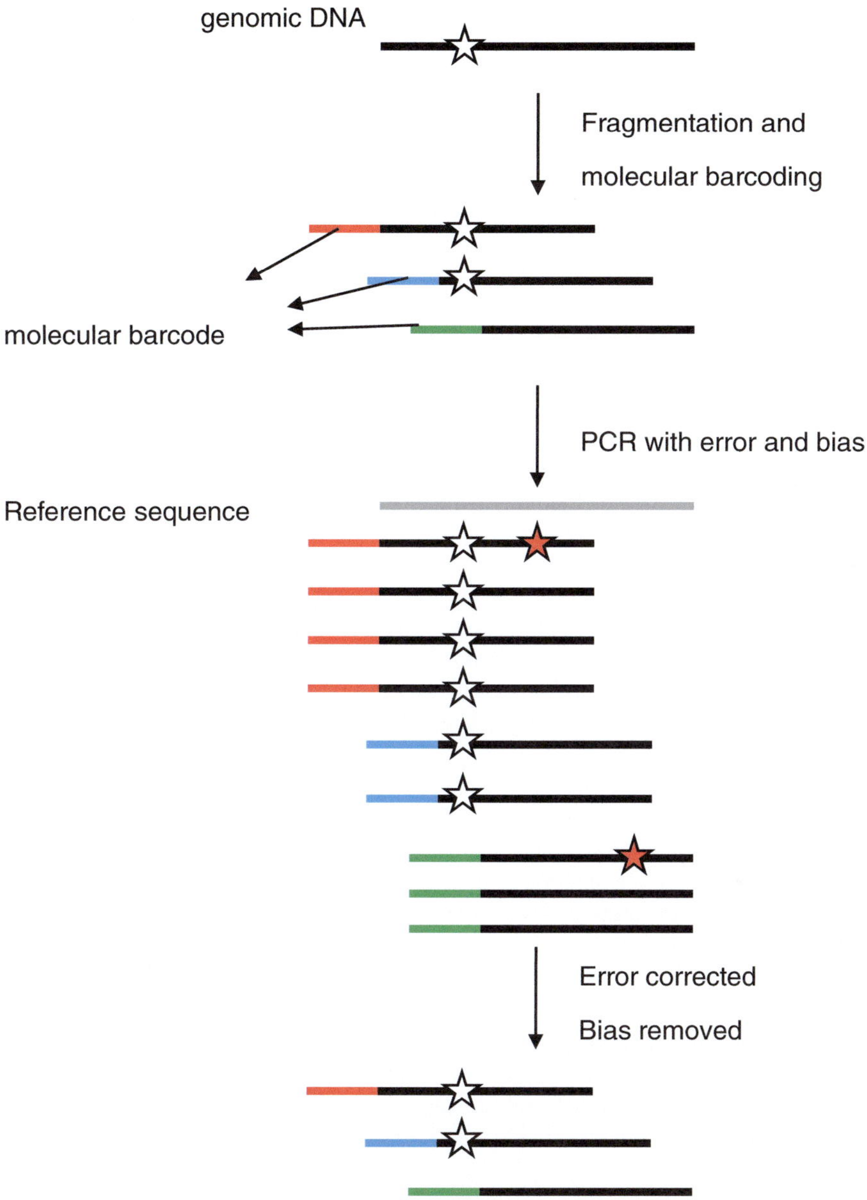

Fig. 5.7 Utilization of molecular barcode. Red, blue, and green bars at the end of the PCR products represent individual molecular barcodes. White and red stars represent a variant in the genome and sequencing error, respectively. Targets are not amplified equally. Because the sequence of PCR products with the same barcode must be identical, sequencing error(s) can be removed by "majority rule." The proportion of the targets in the starting material can be restored by counting the number of reads marked with different barcode

5.4.7 Sequencing of *PMS2*

PMS2CL pseudogene which is highly homologous with exon 9 and 11–15 of *PMS2* makes genetic testing for LS difficult (Fig. 5.1d). Especially exon 12 and 14–15 are almost identical to corresponding exons of *PMS2CL*, it is practically impossible to sequence this region by any of methods described above. In order to analyze this hard-to-read region accurately, long-range PCR is employed using forward primer designed within exon 10 which does not overlap with *PMS2CL* to amplify specifically *PMS2* [30–32]. The PCR product(s) can be sequenced by NGS after fragmentation. It is also possible to perform the second PCR to amplify individual exons and the second PCR products are sequenced. Another approach is to sequence cDNA. This approach should preferentially sequence *PMS2*.

5.5 Interpretation of Variants

Detected variant should be assessed whether the variant causes a disease. The evaluation is based on 1) the amino acid changes expected from the variant, 2) the frequency of the variant in the general population, 3) the evaluation by knowledge databases, 4) the results of the functional analysis of the experiment as the basis for judgment, 5) personal and/or family history of the patient. As for the amino acid changes, it is easy to imagine from the sequence changes, the possibility of splicing abnormalities caused by the variants should not be ignored. Analysis using mRNA is very useful for finding these abnormalities. If the variant's frequency in the general population is sufficiently high (compared to the prevalence of the disease), the variant can be judged not to be pathogenic. It should be noted that the frequencies can vary widely between ethnic groups. Evaluations by knowledge databases such as InSiGHT, ClinVar, HGMD, etc. are also referenced. Since the level of evidence varies with the variant and/or database, it should be used with caution. The results of the functional analysis are mainly based on the literature. Its contents should be carefully reviewed. Based on these criteria, variants are evaluated using guidelines such as ACMG 2015 [1]. InSiGHT has established their own criteria specific to the MMR gene. In any case, it is important to use certain criteria for evaluation. In case of LS, molecular tests, such as MSI testing and IHC, are widely used, but those results are not included in the above criteria. In recent years, evaluation methods that include variant(s) of the MMR genes in tumors and results of IHC have been advocated [2, 3].

5.6 Summary and Perspective

Extensive effort has been made to identify LS patients (family) and variants in LS causative genes. Multigene panel testing using NGS makes it possible to detect single nucleotide variants (SNVs), small indels and copy number variation in the same assay. This will give more chances to diagnose with Lynch syndrome. Their clinical and genetic information should be collected as much as possible and deposit them in the database to use as clinical practice.

References

1. Peltomäki P. Role of DNA mismatch repair defects in the pathogenesis of human cancer. J Clin Oncol. 2003;21:1174–9.
2. Kuiper RP, et al. Recurrence and variability of germline EPCAM deletions in Lynch syndrome. Hum Mutat. 2011;32:407–14.
3. Goel A, et al. De novo constitutional MLH1 epimutations confer early-onset colorectal cancer in two new sporadic Lynch syndrome cases, with derivation of the epimutation on the paternal allele in one. Int J Cancer. 2011;128:869–78.
4. Niessen RC, et al. Germline hypermethylation of MLH1 and EPCAM deletions are a frequent cause of Lynch syndrome. Genes Chromosom Cancer. 2009;48:737–44.
5. Kunkel TA, Erie DA. DNA mismatch repair. Annu Rev Biochem. 2005;74:681–710.
6. Kunkel TA, Erie DA. Eukaryotic mismatch repair in relation to DNA replication. Annu Rev Genet. 2015;49:291–313.
7. Bakry D, et al. Genetic and clinical determinants of constitutional mismatch repair deficiency syndrome: report from the constitutional mismatch repair deficiency consortium. Eur J Cancer. 2014;50:987–96.
8. Nakagawa H, et al. Mismatch repair gene PMS2: disease-causing germline mutations are frequent in patients whose tumors stain negative for PMS2 protein, but paralogous genes obscure mutation detection and interpretation. Cancer Res. 2004;64:4721–7.
9. De Vos M, Hayward BE, Picton S, Sheridan E, Bonthron DT. Novel PMS2 pseudogenes can conceal recessive mutations causing a distinctive childhood cancer syndrome. Am J Hum Genet. 2004;74:954–64.
10. van der Klift HM, et al. Quantification of sequence exchange events between *PMS2* and *PMS2CL* provides a basis for improved mutation scanning of Lynch syndrome patients. Hum Mutat. 2010;31(5):578–87.
11. Hayward BE, et al. Extensive gene conversion at the *PMS2* DNA mismatch repair locus. Hum Mutat. 2007;28:424–30.
12. Taylor NP, et al. MLH3 mutation in endometrial cancer. Cancer Res. 2006;66:7502–8.
13. Adam R, et al. Exome sequencing identifies biallelic MSH3 germline mutations as a recessive subtype of colorectal adenomatous polyposis. Am J Hum Genet. 2016;99:337–51.
14. Espenschied CR, et al. Multigene panel testing provides a new perspective on Lynch syndrome. J Clin Oncol. 2017;35:2568–75.
15. Win AK, et al. Prevalence and penetrance of major genes and polygenes for colorectal cancer. Cancer Epidemiol Biomark Prev. 2017;26:404–12.
16. Vasen HF, Watson P, Mecklin JP, Lynch HT. New clinical criteria for hereditary nonpolyposis colorectal cancer (HNPCC, Lynch syndrome) proposed by the International Collaborative group on HNPCC. Gastroenterology. 1999;116:1453–6.
17. Vasen HF, Mecklin JP, Khan PM, Lynch HT. The International Collaborative Group on Hereditary Non-polyposis Colorectal Cancer (ICG-HNPCC). Dis Colon Rectum. 1991;34:424–5.
18. Umar A, et al. Revised Bethesda guidelines for hereditary nonpolyposis colorectal cancer (Lynch syndrome) and microsatellite instability. J Natl Cancer Inst. 2004;96:261–8.
19. Rodriguez-Bigas MA, et al. A National Cancer Institute Workshop on Hereditary Nonpolyposis Colorectal Cancer Syndrome: meeting highlights and Bethesda guidelines. J Natl Cancer Inst. 1997;89:1758–62.
20. ten Broeke SW, et al. Lynch syndrome caused by germline PMS2 mutations: delineating the cancer risk. J Clin Oncol. 2015;33:319–25.
21. Senter L, et al. The clinical phenotype of Lynch syndrome due to germ-line PMS2 mutations. Gastroenterology. 2008;135:419–428.e1.
22. Li L, et al. Distinct patterns of germ-line deletions inMLH1 andMSH2: the implication of Alu repetitive element in the genetic etiology of Lynch syndrome (HNPCC). Hum Mutat. 2006;27:388.

23. Yamaguchi T, Wakatsuki T, Kikuchi M, Horiguchi S-I, Akagi K. The silent mutation MLH1 c.543C>T resulting in aberrant splicing can cause Lynch syndrome: a case report. Jpn J Clin Oncol. 2017;47:576–80.
24. Nallamilli BRR, Hegde M. Genetic testing for hereditary nonpolyposis colorectal cancer (HNPCC). Curr Protoc Hum Genet. 2017;94:10.12.1–10.12.23.
25. Sikkema-Raddatz B, et al. Targeted next-generation sequencing can replace sanger sequencing in clinical diagnostics. Hum Mutat. 2013;34:1035–42.
26. van Nimwegen KJM, et al. Is the $1000 genome as near as we think? A cost analysis of next-generation sequencing. Clin Chem. 2016;62:1458–64.
27. Mertes F, et al. Targeted enrichment of genomic DNA regions for next-generation sequencing. Brief Funct Genomics. 2011;10:374–86.
28. Peng Q, Vijaya Satya R, Lewis M, Randad P, Wang Y. Reducing amplification artifacts in high multiplex amplicon sequencing by using molecular barcodes. BMC Genomics. 2015;16:589.
29. Chang F, Li MM. Clinical application of amplicon-based next-generation sequencing in cancer. Cancer Genet. 2013;206:413–9.
30. Li J, et al. A comprehensive strategy for accurate mutation detection of the highly homologous PMS2. J Mol Diagn. 2015;17:545–53.
31. Vaughn CP, Hart KJ, Samowitz WS, Swensen JJ. Avoidance of pseudogene interference in the detection of 3′ deletions in PMS2. Hum Mutat. 2011;32:1063–71.
32. Clendenning M, et al. Long-range PCR facilitates the identification of PMS2-specific mutations. Hum Mutat. 2006;27:490–5.

Lynch Syndrome-Associated Gynecological Malignancies

6

Wataru Yamagami and Daisuke Aoki

Abstract

Lynch syndrome-associated gynecological malignancies include endometrial and ovarian cancer. Endometrial cancer is particularly common following colorectal cancer and may be a sentinel cancer. The lifetime incidence of endometrial cancer in patients with Lynch syndrome is 25–60%. Various studies have examined the characteristics and prognosis of Lynch syndrome-associated gynecological malignancies, but there is no consensus. Endometrial cancer is diagnosed by endometrial biopsy, but there is no established surveillance system. Patient education on initial symptoms, routine endometrial biopsy, and transvaginal ultrasonography are performed in clinical practice, but evidence for the efficacy of these methods is limited. The lifetime incidence of ovarian cancer ranges from 4 to 12% and many patients develop epithelial ovarian cancer. Ovarian cancer is initially diagnosed by imaging, with surgery required for definite pathological diagnosis. There is no surveillance system, but patient education, transvaginal ultrasonography, and measurement of serum CA125 are currently used. Prophylactic hysterectomy and bilateral salpingo-oophorectomy are candidates of surgical procedures for preventing Lynch syndrome-associated gynecological malignancies.

Keywords

Endometrial cancer · Ovarian cancer · Prophylactic hysterectomy · Bilateral salpingo-oophorectomy

W. Yamagami (✉) · D. Aoki
Department of Obstetrics and Gynecology,
Keio University School of Medicine, Tokyo, Japan
e-mail: gami@z8.keio.jp; aoki@z7.keio.jp

N. Tomita (ed.), *Lynch Syndrome*, https://doi.org/10.1007/978-981-15-6891-6_6

Table 6.1 Cancer risks by gene individuals with Lynch syndrome age ≤70 years compared to the general population

Cancer type	General population risk (%)	Risk		
		MLH1 and MSH2 (%)	MSH6 (%)	PMS2 (%)
Colorectal	5.5	M:27–74 F: 22–53	M: 22 F: 10	M: 20 F: 15
Endometrial	2.7	14–54	16–26	15
Gastric	<1	0.2–13	M: 6 F: 22	6
Ovarian	1.6	4–20		
Small bowel	<1	4–12		
Hepatobiliary tract	<1	0.2–4		
Urinary tract	<1	0.2–25		
Brain	<1	1–4		
Sebaceous neoplasms	<1	1–9	Unknown	
Pancreas	1.5	0.4–4		
Prostate	16.2	9–30		
Breast	12.4	5–18		

M Male, *F* Female
Cited from reference [1] (modified)

6.1 Introduction

Patients with Lynch syndrome are at risk for developing secondary cancer, including colorectal, endometrial, ovarian, gastric, small intestinal, hepatobiliary, upper urinary tract, skin cancers, and brain tumors (Table 6.1). In these malignant diseases, endometrial and ovarian cancers are gynecological malignancies. In this chapter, the diagnosis and treatment of endometrial and ovarian cancers are reviewed, and surveillance for these cancers in patients with Lynch syndrome is outlined.

6.2 Endometrial Cancer

6.2.1 Characteristics

Most endometrial cancers are sporadic and few are hereditary tumors. The most typical hereditary tumor is Lynch syndrome. In universal screening of 346 patients with endometrial cancer in Japan, 42 had suspected Lynch syndrome and 10 were diagnosed with Lynch syndrome [2]. Women with Lynch syndrome have a high risk of developing endometrial cancer, second only to colorectal cancer (CRC). The incidence of endometrial cancer in patients with Lynch syndrome is 26–60% and the mean onset age is 48–62 years old [1], whereas the lifetime incidence in the general population is 2.7%. Of 315 patients diagnosed with Lynch syndrome, 69

(33%) were diagnosed with endometrial cancer and 17.3% were <40 years old at the time of diagnosis [3].

Endometrial cancer has mutation of MSH6 more often than MLH1 and MSH2 (71% versus 27 and 40%), whereas MLH1 and MSH2 mutations are more common in CRC [4, 5]. Endometrial cancer is considered to be a sentinel cancer of Lynch syndrome, similar to CRC. Microsatellite instability (MSI) is not correlated with the stage, histological type, or myometrial invasion of endometrial cancer, but cases with MSI have a better prognosis than those without MSI [6]. On the other hand, it has also been reported that there is no difference in prognosis between Lynch syndrome-associated and sporadic endometrial cancer [7].

Of women with both CRC and endometrial cancer, 14% were simultaneously diagnosed with the two cancers, 44% developed endometrial or ovarian cancer first, and 42% had CRC first [8]. These results show the importance of gynecologists identifying patients with Lynch syndrome. The interval between CRC diagnosis and development of another Lynch syndrome-related cancer is 8 years (range 1–26 years), whereas a significantly longer time of 11 years (1–39 years) is required for patients with endometrial cancer to develop another cancer [8]. The risks for developing endometrial cancer within 10 years after the development of CRC are estimated to be 23.4% (95% CI: 15–36%) and 1.6% (95% CI: 0.7–3.8%) in patients with and without Lynch syndrome, respectively. The adjusted hazard ratio in the Lynch syndrome group was 6.2 (95% CI: 2.20–17.73) compared with non-Lynch syndrome cases [9].

A comparative study of patients with Lynch syndrome-related and sporadic endometrial cancer in Japan found rates of endometrioid carcinoma of 86% and 97.6%, respectively, indicating a slightly higher incidence of non-endometroid carcinoma in Lynch syndrome-related cancer. However, many cases of well-differentiated endometrioid carcinoma, but no type II endometrial cancer and no significant difference in myometrial invasion, lymphovascular space invasion, or advanced stage have been found in other studies of Lynch syndrome-related cancer. Onset in the lower uterine segment (LUS) is also a feature of Lynch syndrome-related endometrial cancer [10, 11]. The incidence of endometrial cancer in the LUS is 3% in the general population, but 29% in patients with Lynch syndrome associated with MSH2 mutation [12].

6.2.2 Diagnosis

Patients with initial symptoms of endometrial cancer (metrorrhagia, menstrual abnormality, vaginal discharge) and postmenopausal women with endometrial thickness of ≥5 mm on transvaginal ultrasonography undergo endometrial biopsy or total endometrial curettage. If a patient is diagnosed with endometrial cancer, the tumor stage is determined by diagnostic imaging. It is common to perform pelvic magnetic resonance imaging (MRI) to estimate myometrial invasion, cervical stromal invasion, and ovarian metastasis, and then perform chest to pelvic computed tomography (CT) or a positron emission tomography (PET)/CT scan to assess lymph node metastasis and distant metastasis. If a patient cannot be diagnosed with endometrial cancer pathologically, but has prolonged symptoms or abnormal endometrial thickness in transvaginal ultrasonography, a subsidiary diagnosis by hysteroscopy is used to examine if a papillary lesion that may be malignant is present in the uterine cavity.

6.2.3 Treatment

The standard treatment for endometrial cancer is surgical therapy. Standard procedures include hysterectomy, bilateral salpingo-oophorectomy, and retroperitoneal lymph node dissection. If a patient has shallow myometrial invasion and endometrioid carcinoma G1–G2, retroperitoneal lymph node dissection may be omitted. However, a case with deeper myometrial invasion and poorly differentiated cancer (e.g., endometrioid carcinoma G3, serous and clear cell carcinoma) may require dissection of retroperitoneal lymph nodes, including para-aortic lymph nodes and omentectomy. For endometrial cancer in stage I, laparoscopic and robot-assisted surgery can be used. Patients who cannot undergo surgery due to internal complications and age receive radiotherapy. Postoperative treatment for cases with a risk of recurrence includes radiotherapy with extrapelvic irradiation and brachytherapy and chemotherapy with paclitaxel and carboplatin (TC) regimens. For MSI-positive patients with advanced or recurrent endometrial cancer, the addition of anti-PD-1 antibodies to chemotherapy as immune checkpoint inhibitors has been found to be effective. Hormone therapy with medroxyprogesterone acetate (MPA) may be used for progesterone receptor-positive well-differentiated endometrioid carcinoma.

6.2.4 Surveillance

Surveillance for endometrial cancer has not been established due to a lack of sufficient evidence for this approach, in comparison with that for surveillance of CRC. Screening of endometrial cancer is not common in the general population because the morbidity is low and metrorrhagia often occurs at an early stage. However, the onset age of Lynch syndrome-associated endometrial cancer is 10–15 years earlier than the mean diagnostic age of sporadic endometrial cancer and its incidence is high; therefore, there is a need for the design of a surveillance strategy [13].

Most patients with endometrial cancer have early symptoms, including metrorrhagia, postmenopausal bleeding, and vaginal discharge, and women with Lynch syndrome should be given instructions on these symptoms [1]. Endometrial biopsy every 1 or 2 years may be considered, but there is insufficient evidence for the value of this procedure as surveillance [14–16]. For postmenopausal women, the endometrial thickness can be assessed by transvaginal ultrasonography; however, again there is limited evidence. Endometrial thickness obtained from transvaginal ultrasonography is not recommended for assessment in premenopausal women.

There is no evidence that prophylactic hysterectomy improves prognosis, but there is evidence that this procedure decreases the morbidity of endometrial cancer, which makes it a viable option [3]. The appropriate timing of hysterectomy is not determined and the decision should be made based on the status of the patient. Hysterectomy is reasonable for patients with MLH1, PSH2, EPCAM, PMS2, and MSH6 mutations to reduce risks. With regard to conservative therapy, epidemiological studies suggest that the administration of oral contraceptives for 1 year or more to women with MMR gene mutations significantly decreases the risk for endometrial cancer (HR: 0.39, 95% CI: 0.23–0.64) [17]. Women with Lynch syndrome given oral contraceptives for 3 months also have decreased endometrial hyperplasia [18]. However, no prospective intervention study has examined the risk-reducing effect of contraceptives on endometrial cancer.

There are conflicting findings concerning transvaginal ultrasonography and endometrial biopsy. A screening study in 171 Lynch syndrome patients and 98 Lynch syndrome-like patients detected endometrial cancer in two patients based on symptoms who were not detected by transvaginal ultrasonography. Both patients were cured [19]. On the other hand, in a cohort study in Finland of surveillance using endometrial biopsy and transvaginal ultrasonography every 2–3 years, endometrial and ovarian cancers were found in 19 and 6 women, respectively, and no patients died, which indicates the efficacy of surveillance [20].

6.3 Ovarian Cancer

6.3.1 Characteristics

The overall lifetime risk of ovarian cancer is 1.3% in the general population, but women with Lynch syndrome have a much higher lifetime risk of 4–12%. The mean age at diagnosis is 42.5 years, and about 30% of patients with Lynch syndrome-related ovarian cancer are diagnosed at age <30 years, which is younger than for patients with sporadic ovarian cancer. The risks for ovarian cancer are 20% and 24% in women with MLH1 and MSH2 mutations, respectively [21]. Regarding the histological type, almost all cases (94%) are epithelial ovarian cancer, including various tissues similar to nonhereditary ovarian cancer and at a relatively early stage. The rate of ovarian borderline tumor is only 4%, which indicates that this tumor is rarely found in Lynch syndrome [22]. Ovarian cancer is sometimes found as a double cancer with endometrial cancer; however, it is rare that patients with double cancer have Lynch syndrome and many cases of double cancer are sporadic [10]. Many patients with ovarian cancer have gene profiles of germline and somatic mutations of HRD-related genes, including BRCA1 and BRCA2, and only 3% have MMR gene mutations; therefore, few patients with ovarian cancer have Lynch syndrome [23, 24].

6.3.2 Diagnosis

The initial symptoms of ovarian cancer are lower abdominal pain, anorexia, early satiety, and frequent urination, but many patients are often asymptomatic in the early stage. Patients with these symptoms undergo transvaginal ultrasonography and those with ovarian swelling undergo pelvic MRI and chest to pelvic CT scan to examine the characteristics of the ovarian lesion, ascites, peritoneal metastasis, lymph node metastasis, and distal metastasis. Serum tumor markers of CA125, HE4, and CA19-9 are tested and high values indicate suspected ovarian cancer. For patients with ascites, aspiration biopsy cytology can be used to support the diagnosis. Histological diagnosis is commonly performed by surgery.

6.3.3 Treatment

The standard therapy for ovarian cancer is surgery and chemotherapy. The surgical procedures are bilateral salpingo-oophorectomy, hysterectomy, omentectomy, and retroperitoneal lymph node dissection. Tumor resection (primary debulking surgery, PDS) is used for cases of stage II or higher with the dissemination and metastatic lesions in the pelvis and peritoneal cavity not to remain gross lesions. Adjuvant therapy includes chemotherapy with TC therapy and the use of molecular targeted drugs, including the angiogenesis inhibitor bevacizumab and the poly(ADP-ribose) polymerase (PARP) inhibitors olaparib, niraparib, and rucaparib. Some patients with advanced cancer who cannot undergo surgery or with lesions that cannot be controlled by surgery are treated with neoadjuvant chemotherapy, and tumor resection (interval debulking surgery, IDS) is recommended after tumor reduction.

6.3.4 Surveillance

There is insufficient evidence for ovarian cancer screening as surveillance in women with Lynch syndrome. The biological characteristics of ovarian cancer in patients with Lynch syndrome differ greatly from those in patients with hereditary breast and ovarian cancer (HBOC). Therefore, surveillance for HBOC does not clearly apply to Lynch syndrome. Women with Lynch syndrome should be informed of ovarian cancer-related symptoms, including acute lower abdominal pain, bloating, increased waist circumference, anorexia, early satiety, and frequent urination [1]. Ovarian cancer screening using serum CA125 and transvaginal ultrasonography does not give enough evidence for other hereditary tumors, including in women with HBOC who have BRCA1 and BRCA2 mutations; however, this screening may be performed for women with Lynch syndrome at the discretion of the physician [25]. Bilateral salpingo-oophorectomy reduces the incidence of ovarian cancer; however, the decision to perform a risk-reducing surgery and the timing of this surgery depends on the patient's status. There is insufficient evidence for the performance of risk-reducing salpingo-oophorectomy (RRSO) in patients with MSH6 or PMS2 mutation [3].

6.4 Reproductive Age

Women of reproductive age with Lynch syndrome would be advised on prenatal diagnosis and assisted reproductive technology, including preimplantation genetic diagnosis. Ethical considerations in different countries and regions also require discussion. A partner of a carrier of allogeneic MMR and EPCAM genes should be informed of the risks for constitutional MMR deficiency (CMMRD).

References

1. Kohlmann W, Gruber S. Lynch syndrome. GeneReviews at GeneTests: medical genetic information resource; 2014. Available at https://www.ncbi.nlm.nih.gov/books/NBK1211/
2. Takahashi K, Sato N, Sugawara T, Kato A, Sato T, Shimizu D, Tamura D, Kito M, Makino K, Shirasawa H, Miura H, Sato W, Kumazawa Y, Sato A, Terada Y. Clinical characteristics of Lynch-like cases collaterally classified by Lynch syndrome identification strategy using universal screening in endometrial cancer. Gynecol Oncol. 2017;147(2):388–95.
3. Schmeler KM, Lynch HT, Chen LM, Munsell MF, Soliman PT, Clark MB, Daniels MS, White KG, Boyd-Rogers SG, Conrad PG, Yang KY, Rubin MM, Sun CC, Slomovitz BM, Gershenson DM, Lu KH. Prophylactic surgery to reduce the risk of gynecologic cancers in the Lynch syndrome. N Engl J Med. 2006;354(3):261–9.
4. Watson P, Vasen HFA, Mecklin JP, Bernstein I, Aarnio M, Järvinen HJ, Myrhøj T, Sunde L, Wijnen JT, Lynch HT. The risk of extra-colonic, extra-endometrial cancer in the Lynch syndrome. Int J Cancer. 2008;123(2):444–9.
5. Vasen HF, Möslein G, Alonso A, Bernstein I, Bertario L, Blanco I, Burn J, Capella G, Engel C, Frayling I, Friedl W, Hes FJ, Hodgson S, Mecklin JP, Møller P, Nagengast F, Parc Y, Renkonen-Sinisalo L, Sampson JR, Stormorken A, Wijnen J. Guidelines for the clinical management of Lynch syndrome (hereditary non-polyposis cancer). J Med Genet. 2007;44(6):353–62.
6. Maxwell GL, Risinger JI, Alvarez AA, Barrett JC, Berchuck A. Favorable survival associated with microsatellite instability in endometrioid endometrial cancers. Obstet Gynecol. 2001;97(3):417–22.
7. Boks DE, Trujillo AP, Voogd AC, Morreau H, Kenter GG, Vasen HF. Survival analysis of endometrial carcinoma associated with hereditary nonpolyposis colorectal cancer. Int J Cancer. 2002;102:198–200.
8. Lu KH, Dinh M, Kohlmann W, Broaddus RR. Gynecologic cancer as a "sentinel cancer" for women with hereditary nonpolyposis colorectal cancer syndrome. Obstet Gynecol. 2005;105(3):569–74.
9. Obermair A, Youlden DR, Young JP, Lindor NM, Baron JA, Newcomb P, Parry S, Hopper JL, Haile R, Jenkins MA. Risk of endometrial cancer for women diagnosed with HNPCC-related colorectal carcinoma. Int J Cancer. 2010;127(11):2678–84.
10. Hirai Y, Banno K, Suzuki M, Ichikawa Y, Udagawa Y, Sugano K, Miki Y. Molecularepidemiological and mutational analysis of DNA mismatch repair (MMR) genes in endometrial cancer patients with HNPCC-associated familial predisposition to cancer. Cancer Sci. 2008;99(9):1715–9.
11. 小西ら 日産婦誌2009 1540-1542

12. Westin SN, Lacour RA, Urbauer DL, Luthra R, Bodurka DC, Lu KH, Broaddus RR. Carcinoma of the lower uterine segment: a newly described association with Lynch syndrome. J Clin Oncol. 2008;26(36):5965–71.
13. Committee on Practice Bulletins-Gynecology, Society of Gynecologic Oncology. ACOG practice bulletin no. 147: Lynch syndrome. Obstet Gynecol. 2014;124(5):1042–54.
14. Dove-Edwin I, Boks D, Goff S, Kenter GG, Carpenter R, Vasen HF, et al. The outcome of endometrial carcinoma surveillance by ultrasound scan in women at risk of hereditary nonpolyposis colorectal carcinoma and familial colorectal carcinoma. Cancer. 2002;94:1708–12.
15. Renkonen-Sinisalo L, Butzow R, Leminen A, Lehtovirta P, Mecklin JP, Jarvinen HJ. Surveillance for endometrial cancer in hereditary nonpolyposis colorectal cancer syndrome. Int J Cancer. 2007;120:821–4.
16. Gerritzen LH, Hoogerbrugge N, Oei AL, Nagengast FM, van Ham MA, Massuger LF, et al. Improvement of endometrial biopsy over transvaginal ultrasound alone for endometrial surveillance in women with Lynch syndrome. Familial Cancer. 2009;8:391–7.
17. Dashti SG, Chau R, Ouakrim DA, Buchanan DD, Clendenning M, Young JP, Winship IM, Arnold J, Ahnen DJ, Haile RW, Casey G, Gallinger S, Thibodeau SN, Lindor NM, Le Marchand L, Newcomb PA, Potter JD, Baron JA, Hopper JL, Jenkins MA, Win AK. Female hormonal factors and the risk of endometrial cancer in lynch syndrome. JAMA. 2015;314(1):61–71.
18. Lu KH, Loose DS, Yates MS, Nogueras-Gonzalez GM, Munsell MF, Chen LM, Lynch H, Cornelison T, Boyd-Rogers S, Rubin M, Daniels MS, Conrad P, Milbourne A, Gershenson DM, Broaddus RR. Prospective multicenter randomized intermediate biomarker study of oral contraceptive versus depo-provera for prevention of endometrial cancer in women with Lynch syndrome. Cancer Prev Res (Phila). 2013;6:774–81.
19. Dove-Edwin I, Boks D, Goff S, Kenter GG, Carpenter R, Vasen HF, Thomas HJ. The outcome of endometrial carcinoma surveillance by ultrasound scan in women at risk of hereditary nonpolyposis colorectal carcinoma and familial colorectal carcinoma. Cancer. 2002;94(6):1708–12.
20. Järvinen HJ, Renkonen-Sinisalo L, Aktán-Collán K, Peltomäki P, Aaltonen LA, Mecklin JP. Ten years after mutation testing for Lynch syndrome: cancer incidence and outcome in mutation-positive and mutation-negative family members. J Clin Oncol. 2009;27(28):4793–7.
21. Bonadona V, Bonaïti B, Olschwang S, Grandjouan S, Huiart L, Longy M, Guimbaud R, Buecher B, Bignon YJ, Caron O, Colas C, Noguès C, Lejeune-Dumoulin S, Olivier-Faivre L, Polycarpe-Osaer F, Nguyen TD, Desseigne F, Saurin JC, Berthet P, Leroux D, Duffour J, Manouvrier S, Frébourg T, Sobol H, Lasset C, Bonaïti-Pellié C, French Cancer Genetics Network. Cancer risks associated with germline mutations in MLH1, MSH2, and MSH6 genes in Lynch syndrome. JAMA. 2011;305(22):2304–10.
22. Watson P, Bützow R, Lynch HT, Mecklin JP, Järvinen HJ, Vasen HF, Madlensky L, Fidalgo P, Bernstein I, International Collaborative Group on HNPCC. The clinical features of ovarian cancer in hereditary nonpolyposis colorectal cancer. Gynecol Oncol. 2001;82(2):223–8.
23. Konstantinopoulos PA, Ceccaldi R, Shapiro GI, D'Andrea AD. Homologous recombination deficiency: exploiting the fundamental vulnerability of ovarian cancer. Cancer Discov. 2015;5(11):1137–54.
24. Hirasawa A, Imoto I, Naruto T, Akahane T, Yamagami W, Nomura H, Masuda K, Susumu N, Tsuda H, Aoki D. Prevalence of pathogenic germline variants detected by multigene sequencing in unselected Japanese patients with ovarian cancer. Oncotarget. 2017;8(68):112258–67.
25. Evans DG, Gaarenstroom KN, Stirling D, Shenton A, Maehle L, Dørum A, Steel M, Lalloo F, Apold J, Porteous ME, Vasen HF, van Asperen CJ, Moller P. Screening for familial ovarian cancer: poor survival of BRCA1/2 related cancers. J Med Genet. 2009;46(9):593–7.

Lynch Syndrome-Associated Urological Malignancies

7

Hisashi Hasumi and Masahiro Yao

Abstract

Lynch syndrome is a hereditary cancer syndrome caused by germline alterations in mismatch repair (MMR) genes. Recently, there is growing evidence of an increased risk of development of upper tract urothelial carcinomas (UTUC) in Lynch syndrome and in fact, upper tract urothelial carcinoma has been found to be the third most common Lynch-associated malignancy. Interestingly, universal screening of UTUC exhibited that 5% of UTUC is Lynch-associated, highlighting the importance of medical and family history of UTUC patients. Several studies have suggested that Lynch patients may have an increased risk of development of bladder and prostate cancer; however, this potential association may need further investigations because of the high incidence of those cancers in general population.

Keywords

Lynch syndrome · Upper tract urothelial carcinoma (UTUC) · Mismatch repair (MMR) genes · MSH2 · MSH6

7.1 Introduction

Lynch syndrome is a cancer predisposition syndrome caused by germline alterations in mismatch repair (MMR) genes, including *MSH2*, *MLH1*, *MSH6*, and *PMS2*, or by germline deletions affecting the 3′ exon of *EPCAM* gene resulting in epigenetic silencing of the downstream MSH2 locus by promoter hypermethylation [1, 2]. Lynch syndrome predisposes affected patients to develop most frequently colon cancer, and in addition to colon cancer, extra-colonic tumor spectrum of Lynch

H. Hasumi (✉) · M. Yao
Department of Urology, Yokohama City University, Yokohama, Japan
e-mail: hasumi@yokohama-cu.ac.jp

N. Tomita (ed.), *Lynch Syndrome*, https://doi.org/10.1007/978-981-15-6891-6_7

syndrome has been reported which includes endometrial, ovarian, urothelial, gastric, small bowel, pancreatic, hepatobiliary, brain, and sebaceous neoplasm [3–6]. The study of 121 Lynch syndrome families exhibited that the overall cumulative lifetime risk of developing an extra-colonic neoplasm was 37.5 (95% CI: 34.0–40.1) [4]. Among Lynch-associated extra-colonic neoplasms, upper tract urothelial carcinoma (UTUC) has been found to be the third most common Lynch-associated malignancy. In addition, several reports suggest the potential link between Lynch syndrome and bladder or prostate cancer. Here, we describe how to manage Lynch syndrome-associated urological malignancies as well as how to identify Lynch patients from upper tract urothelial carcinomas developed in general population.

7.2 Upper Tract Urothelial Carcinoma (UTUC) Development in Lynch Syndrome

Although upper tract urothelial carcinoma (UTUC) is a relatively rare disease accounting for around 5% of all urological malignancies, UTUC is the third most common Lynch-associated malignancy, accounting for 5% of Lynch-associated malignancies, after colonic (63%) and endometrial (9%) neoplasms [7–9]. Because UTUC clinically tends to present an aggressive form of urothelial carcinoma with higher stage and higher grade compared to bladder cancer, an early detection is a key for the better management of Lynch-associated UTUC [10, 11]. Considering a limited sensitivity of urinary cytology test and a patient's physical burden from retrograde pyelography or ureteroscope, combination of urinary analysis and computed tomography is currently a valid screening method for the early detection of Lynch-associated UTUC [12].

Interestingly, universal screening of UTUC exhibited loss of mismatch repair proteins including, MSH2 and MSH6, in 5.0–11.3% of universally screened UTUC cases, suggesting that loss of MMR genes may be a critical driver for tumorigenesis in a subset of UTUC [9, 13, 14]. Of note, germline alterations in MMR genes were found in about 5% in universally screened UTUC cases, indicating that the considerable number of Lynch-associated UTUC cases may be overlooked in medical practices. The majority (64%) of patients with Lynch-associated UTUC have previous history of an additional Lynch-associated cancer, most commonly colorectal carcinoma [13]. Therefore, urologists should carefully obtain a medical and family history of Lynch-associated malignancies from patients with UTUC and consider further screening tests of Lynch syndrome for UTUC cases suspected for Lynch syndrome.

Two clinicopathologic criteria, i.e., Amsterdam criteria and revised Bethesda criteria, can be used for identification of individuals at risk of Lynch syndrome; however, these criteria are designed to identify Lynch patients mainly from colon cancer, thereby have a limited efficacy to identify Lynch patients from extra-colonic cancers [15]. An average age of Lynch-associated UTUC is 64 years whereas that of overall UTUC is 70 years, and Lynch-associated UTUC often lacks the typical risk factors associated with urothelial carcinomas such as smoking [13]. Histologically, Lynch-associated UTUC exhibits patterns of inverted growth, increased intra-tumoral lymphocytes, and the presence of pushing tumor/stromal interface [9, 13]. These clinicopathologic characteristics may be useful for considering further screening tests for Lynch syndrome.

Since the loss of MMR genes leads to the defective correction of DNA replication errors, microsatellites instability (MSI) can be used as a marker of Lynch syndrome [1]. However, MSI in Lynch-associated extra-colonic cancers is not fully assessed, whereas MSI in Lynch-associated colon cancer is well validated [14, 16–18]. In fact, a subset of Lynch-associated UTUC may be MSI stable [14]. For this reason, immunohistochemistry (IHC) of MMR genes is broadly used as a useful screening test for Lynch-associated UTUC. The definitive diagnosis of Lynch syndrome requires genetic testing of MMR genes.

7.3 Possible Link Between Lynch Syndrome and Bladder Cancer

The incidence of bladder cancer in Lynch syndrome remains controversial mainly because of the high incidence of those tumors in the general population [15, 19–21]. However, there are several reports regarding an increased risk of development of bladder cancer in Lynch syndrome. According to the previous report, 6.2% of MSH2 mutation carriers developed bladder cancer [21]. Because prior or concurrent UTUC may confound results as a result of seeding in the bladder, the incidence of bladder cancer in Lynch syndrome should be carefully assessed with further studies [15].

7.4 Possible Link Between Lynch Syndrome and Prostate Cancer

Recent reports suggested the potential link between prostate cancer and Lynch syndrome. Integration of publically available database revealed that the estimated risk of development of prostate cancer is 2.28 (95% CI, 1.37–3.19) for all men from MMR mutation-carrying families [22]. In addition, the cumulative risk of prostate cancer at age of 70 was 3.7% (95% CI: 2.3–4.9) in Danish 288 Lynch syndrome families and the other group showed that a standardized rate ratio of prostate cancer was 4.87 (95% CI: 2.43–8.71) with 188 Lynch males [23, 24]. Because PSA is an accessible marker for early detection of prostate cancer, a periodic surveillance of PSA may be recommended for patients with Lynch syndrome.

7.5 High MSI of Chemotherapy Resistant Testicular Cancer

Testicular cancer is rare compared to other urological malignancies such as bladder cancer and prostate cancer. To date, there has been no report regarding an association of testicular cancer with Lynch syndrome. However, because a proportion of chemotherapy resistant testicular cancers exhibits high MSI, IHC of MMR proteins and MSI testing may be considered for chemotherapy-resistant testicular cancers [25].

7.6 Conclusion

UTUC is developed in 5% of Lynch patients, which is the third common malignancy in Lynch syndrome. Several studies indicate the link between Lynch syndrome and other urological malignancies including bladder cancer and prostate cancer. Urologists should be aware of Lynch-associated UTUC and consider screening tests with UTUC cases suspected for Lynch syndrome.

References

1. Baretti M, Le DT. DNA mismatch repair in cancer. Pharmacol Ther. 2018;189:45–62.
2. Ligtenberg MJ, Kuiper RP, Chan TL, Goossens M, Hebeda KM, Voorendt M, Lee TY, Bodmer D, Hoenselaar E, Hendriks-Cornelissen SJ, et al. Heritable somatic methylation and inactivation of MSH2 in families with Lynch syndrome due to deletion of the 3′ exons of TACSTD1. Nat Genet. 2009;41:112–7.
3. Bonis PA, Trikalinos TA, Chung M, Chew P, Ip S, DeVine DA, Lau J. Hereditary nonpolyposis colorectal cancer: diagnostic strategies and their implications. Evid Rep Technol Assess (Full Rep). 2007:1–180.
4. Barrow E, Robinson L, Alduaij W, Shenton A, Clancy T, Lalloo F, Hill J, Evans DG. Cumulative lifetime incidence of extracolonic cancers in Lynch syndrome: a report of 121 families with proven mutations. Clin Genet. 2009;75:141–9.
5. Watson P, Riley B. The tumor spectrum in the Lynch syndrome. Familial Cancer. 2005;4:245–8.
6. Watson P, Vasen HFA, Mecklin JP, Bernstein I, Aarnio M, Jarvinen HJ, Myrhoj T, Sunde L, Wijnen JT, Lynch HT. The risk of extra-colonic, extra-endometrial cancer in the Lynch syndrome. Int J Cancer. 2008;123:444–9.
7. Roupret M, Yates DR, Comperat E, Cussenot O. Upper urinary tract urothelial cell carcinomas and other urological malignancies involved in the hereditary nonpolyposis colorectal cancer (lynch syndrome) tumor spectrum. Eur Urol. 2008;54:1226–36.
8. Barrow PJ, Ingham S, O'Hara C, Green K, McIntyre I, Lalloo F, Hill J, Evans DG. The spectrum of urological malignancy in Lynch syndrome. Familial Cancer. 2013;12:57–63.
9. Urakami S, Inoshita N, Oka S, Miyama Y, Nomura S, Arai M, Sakaguchi K, Kurosawa K, Okaneya T. Clinicopathological characteristics of patients with upper urinary tract urothelial cancer with loss of immunohistochemical expression of the DNA mismatch repair proteins in universal screening. Int J Urol. 2018;25:151–6.
10. Blaszyk H, Wang L, Dietmaier W, Hofstadter F, Burgart LJ, Cheville JC, Hartmann A. Upper tract urothelial carcinoma: a clinicopathologic study including microsatellite instability analysis. Mod Pathol. 2002;15:790–7.
11. Zhang B, Yu W, Feng X, Zhao Z, Fan Y, Meng Y, Hu S, Cui Y, He Q, Zhang H, et al. Prognostic significance of PD-L1 expression on tumor cells and tumor-infiltrating mononuclear cells in upper tract urothelial carcinoma. Med Oncol. 2017;34:94.
12. Myrhoj T, Andersen MB, Bernstein I. Screening for urinary tract cancer with urine cytology in Lynch syndrome and familial colorectal cancer. Familial Cancer. 2008;7:303–7.
13. Harper HL, McKenney JK, Heald B, Stephenson A, Campbell SC, Plesec T, Magi-Galluzzi C. Upper tract urothelial carcinomas: frequency of association with mismatch repair protein loss and lynch syndrome. Mod Pathol. 2017;30:146–56.
14. Metcalfe MJ, Petros FG, Rao P, Mork ME, Xiao L, Broaddus RR, Matin SF. Universal point of care testing for Lynch syndrome in patients with upper tract urothelial carcinoma. J Urol. 2018;199:60–5.
15. Huang D, Matin SF, Lawrentschuk N, Roupret M. Systematic review: an update on the spectrum of urological malignancies in Lynch syndrome. Bladder Cancer. 2018;4:261–8.

16. Kuismanen SA, Moisio AL, Schweizer P, Truninger K, Salovaara R, Arola J, Butzow R, Jiricny J, Nystrom-Lahti M, Peltomaki P. Endometrial and colorectal tumors from patients with hereditary nonpolyposis colon cancer display different patterns of microsatellite instability. Am J Pathol. 2002;160:1953–8.
17. Hause RJ, Pritchard CC, Shendure J, Salipante SJ. Classification and characterization of microsatellite instability across 18 cancer types. Nat Med. 2016;22:1342–50.
18. Mork M, Hubosky SG, Roupret M, Margulis V, Raman J, Lotan Y, O'Brien T, You N, Shariat SF, Matin SF. Lynch syndrome: a primer for urologists and panel recommendations. J Urol. 2015;194:21–9.
19. Win AK, Lindor NM, Young JP, Macrae FA, Young GP, Williamson E, Parry S, Goldblatt J, Lipton L, Winship I, et al. Risks of primary extracolonic cancers following colorectal cancer in lynch syndrome. J Natl Cancer Inst. 2012;104:1363–72.
20. Joost P, Therkildsen C, Dominguez-Valentin M, Jonsson M, Nilbert M. Urinary tract cancer in Lynch syndrome; increased risk in carriers of MSH2 mutations. Urology. 2015;86:1212–7.
21. Skeldon SC, Semotiuk K, Aronson M, Holter S, Gallinger S, Pollett A, Kuk C, van Rhijn B, Bostrom P, Cohen Z, et al. Patients with Lynch syndrome mismatch repair gene mutations are at higher risk for not only upper tract urothelial cancer but also bladder cancer. Eur Urol. 2013;63:379–85.
22. Ryan S, Jenkins MA, Win AK. Risk of prostate cancer in Lynch syndrome: a systematic review and meta-analysis. Cancer Epidemiol Biomark Prev. 2014;23:437–49.
23. Dominguez-Valentin M, Joost P, Therkildsen C, Jonsson M, Rambech E, Nilbert M. Frequent mismatch-repair defects link prostate cancer to Lynch syndrome. BMC Urol. 2016;16:15.
24. Haraldsdottir S, Hampel H, Wei L, Wu C, Frankel W, Bekaii-Saab T, de la Chapelle A, Goldberg RM. Prostate cancer incidence in males with Lynch syndrome. Genet Med. 2014;16:553–7.
25. Mayer F, Wermann H, Albers P, Stoop H, Gillis AJ, Hartmann JT, Bokemeyer CC, Oosterhuis JW, Looijenga LH, Honecker F. Histopathological and molecular features of late relapses in non-seminomas. BJU Int. 2011;107:936–43.

Screening for Lynch Syndrome

8

Tatsuro Yamaguchi

Abstract

To date, various testings to screen for Lynch syndrome have been proposed. Classically, Amsterdam criteria I/II and Bethesda guideline were developed as clinical screening testing using family history and cancer history. Since these screening testings do not detect all colorectal cancer with microsatellite instability, the universal tumor screening for Lynch syndrome using microsatellite instability testing or immunohistochemistry of mismatch repair proteins in all colorectal cancer and endometrial cancer is recommended. The effectiveness of immunohistochemical analysis of the mismatch repair proteins is similar to that of microsatellite instability; however, immunohistochemistry is more readily available and helps to direct gene testing. The universal genetic testing is reported from some groups; however, it is still premature to generalize the universal genetic testing as a screening test for Lynch syndrome.

Keywords

Lynch syndrome · Mismatch repair genes · Microsatellite instability · Amsterdam criteria II · Revised Bethesda guidelines · Universal tumor screening

---

T. Yamaguchi (✉)
Department of Clinical Genetics, Tokyo Metropolitan Cancer and Infectious Diseases Center Komagome Hospital, Tokyo, Japan
e-mail: tatsuro@yamaguchi.email.ne.jp

N. Tomita (ed.), *Lynch Syndrome*, https://doi.org/10.1007/978-981-15-6891-6_8

8.1 Introduction

Lynch syndrome, formerly referred to as HNPCC (hereditary non-polyposis colorectal cancer), is an autosomal dominant inheritance caused by germline mutation on mismatch repair genes, including *MLH1*, *MSH2*, *MSH6*, and *PMS2*, and is one of the most common hereditary tumor syndromes, accounting for 1–5% of colorectal cancer patients and affecting 1 out of every 279 individuals worldwide [1]. Lifetime risk for malignant tumor is estimated to be 90% at the age of 80 years old, and half of their kindred, affected Lynch syndrome, are also in high-risk group. Therefore, in order to provide the appropriate surveillance program to Lynch syndrome patients, screening for Lynch syndrome patients is quite important things. Herein, we reviewed various screening methods for Lynch syndrome.

8.2 Clinical Testing

8.2.1 Amsterdam Criteria I and II

The first clinical screening criteria for the identification of Lynch syndrome were developed by the International Collaborative group on HNPCC in 1990 [2]. The criteria came to be called the Amsterdam criteria I after the place name where the meeting was held. The Amsterdam criteria I were known as the "3–2–1 Rule:" three relatives with colorectal cancer, one a first-degree relative of the other two; two successive generations affected; one diagnosed before the age of 50 years. At that time when the Amsterdam criteria I were developed, the causative genes of Lynch syndrome were not detected yet. As a result that mismatch repair genes were identified as causative genes of Lynch syndrome one after another since 1993 [3–5], it had been reported that some families with germline mismatch pathogenic variant do not meet the Amsterdam criteria I or some families met the Amsterdam criteria I were not detected germline mismatch pathogenic variant. Moreover, when the clinical characteristics of Lynch syndrome became increasingly evident, it became to be pointed out that the criteria excluded some Lynch syndrome families because of not taking into account the extracolonic cancers, such as endometrial cancer, small bowel cancer, and ureter and renal pelvic cancer. Therefore, the revised Amsterdam criteria (Amsterdam criteria II) were proposed as new clinical screening criteria for the identification of Lynch syndrome by the International Collaborative group on HNPCC in 1998 [6]. According to the Amsterdam criteria II, Lynch syndrome should be screened the kindred that meets all of the following criteria: (1) the kindred have at least three relatives with an Lynch syndrome-associated cancer (colorectal, endometrial, small bowel, and ureter and renal pelvis cancers), (2) one should be a first-degree relative of the other two, (3) at least two successive generations should be affected, (4) at least one should be diagnosed before age 50, (5) familial adenomatous polyposis should be excluded in the colorectal cancer case(s) if any, (6) tumors should be verified by pathological examination. Both the Amsterdam criteria I and the Amsterdam criteria II should not be used as diagnostic criteria, because these are screening criteria but not diagnostic criteria.

8.2.2 The Bethesda Guidelines and the Revised Bethesda Guidelines

To identify potential Lynch syndrome patients who are not identified by the Amsterdam Criteria I, the Bethesda guidelines were developed for the identification of tumors that should be tested for MSI [7]. Elements of the Bethesda Guidelines include both criteria for assessing colorectal cancer patterns in families meeting the Amsterdam Criteria I and several other characteristics reported more frequently in Lynch syndrome.

In 2004, the Bethesda guidelines were revised to clarify several issues, such as sensitivity-specificity and cost-effectiveness [8]. According to the revised Bethesda Guidelines, the individuals meet the following criteria should be tested MSI: (1) colorectal cancer diagnosed in a patient who is less than 50 years of age, (2) presence of synchronous, metachronous Lynch syndrome-associated tumors (colorectal, endometrial, stomach, small bowel, ovarian, pancreas, ureter and renal pelvis and biliary tract cancers, brain tumors, and sebaceous gland adenomas and keratoacanthomas), regardless of age, (3) colorectal cancer with the MSI-H histology (tumor infiltrating lymphocytes, Crohn's-like lymphocytic reaction, mucinous/signet-ring differentiation, or medullary growth pattern) diagnosed in a patient who is less than 60 years of age, (4) colorectal cancer diagnosed in one or more first-degree relatives with an Lynch syndrome-associated tumor, with one of the cancers being diagnosed under age 50 years, (5) colorectal cancer diagnosed in two or more first- or second-degree relatives with Lynch syndrome-associated tumors, regardless of age. While 27–41% [9] of Lynch syndrome families meet the Amsterdam criteria II [10], 68–89% meet the revised Bethesda guidelines [8]. Thus, more patients with Lynch syndrome can be identified using the revised Bethesda guidelines [9].

8.2.3 Jerusalem Recommendations

To develop consensus for the optimal management of Lynch syndrome and to identify areas of research with the potential to advance the clinical management of Lynch syndrome, the Jerusalem workshop was held on October 2009 [11]. It was pointed out that since many Lynch syndrome patients did not have sufficient family history data from which to construct adequate pedigrees, even the revised Bethesda guidelines were reported not to detect all colorectal cancer with microsatellite instability. Therefore, in the conclusion of the workshop, they recommended that all CRC patients <70 years old should be tested using immunohistochemistry for the four DNA mismatch repair gene products, or alternatively, MSI. Pooled analysis of four large cohorts demonstrated that adding elderly patients who meet the Bethesda guidelines to patients who meet the Jerusalem recommendation as recommended patients for MMR testing increases the sensitivity of diagnosis with Lynch syndrome [9].

8.2.4 Universal Tumor Screening

The universal tumor screening for Lynch syndrome using microsatellite instability testing or immunohistochemistry of mismatch repair proteins in all colorectal cancer and endometrial cancer is recommended by various societies, including Evaluation of genetic applications in practice and prevention [12], National Comprehensive Cancer Network, US Multi-society Task Force on colorectal cancer [13–16], Society for Gynecologic Oncology [17], American College of Obstetrics and Gynecology [18], and Healthy People 2020 goal [19]. As a result of universal tumor screening, 2.8% of colorectal cancer patients were reported to be detected pathogenic variant in MMR genes [20]. However, even universal tumor screening miss individuals who are Lynch syndrome, because neither immunohistochemistry nor microsatellite instability is not perfect [12]. Incremental cost-effectiveness ratio for universal tumor screening for Lynch syndrome was estimated to be $31,391 per year of life saved [21]. As experts agree that interventions with an incremental cost-effectiveness ratio < $50,000 per year of life saved are cost-effective, the universal tumor screening for Lynch syndrome is acceptable in the point of economical view [22].

8.3 Tumor Testing

8.3.1 Microsatellite Instability

A characteristic of microsatellite instability is an accumulation of replication errors, caused by deficiency of mismatch repair system, at microsatellite region in tumor DNA. Thus, microsatellite instability testing compares allelic sizes of microsatellite regions in normal DNA with those in tumor DNA. Classically, five microsatellite markers panel, known as the National Cancer Institute Panel (BAT-25, BAT-26, D2S123, D5S346, and D17S250), is recommended to be used for evaluation of microsatellite instability [7, 23]. However, quasimonomorphic mononucleotide repeats were proven to be high sensitivity and high specificity without corresponding normal DNA [24–26], because it is rare that out of the quasimonomorphic variant range in normal DNA [27].

It was reported that a clear recommendation for the uniform use of a panel of ten microsatellites and a definition of at least 40% instability (using these defined marker loci) in the diagnostic analysis of MSI [28]. Moreover, Both Pentaplex Panel (BAT-25, BAT-26, NR-21, NR-24, and NR-27) and Promega Panel (BAT-25, BAT-26, NR-21, NR-24, and MONO-27) are reported to be higher sensitivity and specificity than NCI panel [26, 29].

Table 8.1 The immunohistochemical expression pattern of the mismatch repair proteins and suspected causative genes

		Proteins			
		MLH1	MSH2	MSH6	PMS2
Genes	*MLH1*	–	+	+	–
	MSH2	+	–	–	+
	MSH6	+	+	–	+
	PMS2	+	+	+	–

8.3.2 Immunohistochemistry Staining

Immunohistochemistry staining test for Lynch syndrome evaluates expressions of four MMR proteins in the tumor. Table 8.1 shows immunohistochemical expression patterns of the mismatch repair proteins and suspected causative genes. MLH1 and PMS2 form a heterodimer, and MSH2 and MSH6 also form a heterodimer. PMS2 only dimerizes with MLH1, while MLH1 forms heterodimers with other mismatch repair proteins as well as PMS2. Similarly, MSH6 only dimerizes with MSH2, while MSH2 forms heterodimers with other mismatch repair proteins as well as MSH6. Therefore, gene mutation and loss of MLH1 and MSH2 invariably result in the degradation of PMS2 and MSH6, respectively, but the converse is not true [30]. The effectiveness of screening with immunohistochemical analysis of the mismatch repair proteins would be similar to that of the more complex strategy of genotyping for microsatellite instability [20]; however, immunohistochemistry is more readily available and helps to direct gene testing [31].

8.3.3 Universal Genetic Testing

Most of tumor developed in Lynch syndrome patients demonstrate microsatellite instability and/or mismatch repair deficiency; however, either testing is not perfect. Moreira and colleague reported that germline mismatch repair gene mutation was detected 12 of 1395 colorectal cancer patients without mismatch repair deficiency from pooled analysis data of 4 large cohorts [9]. A study of universal genetic testing for Lynch syndrome estimated to be 2.2% of colorectal cancer patients being Lynch syndrome [20]. However, the incremental cost-effectiveness ratio for genetic testing was reported to be more than $1,000,000 per year of life saved [21]. Therefore, it is still premature to generalize the universal genetic testing as a screening test for Lynch syndrome.

8.4 Prediction Models

Lynch syndrome prediction models using cancer history data from the patients and their relatives were proposed one after another in 2006 [32–34] (Table 8.2).

Table 8.2 Uniform resource locator of prediction models for Lynch syndrome

Prediction model	Uniform resource locator
MMRpredict [32]	http://hnpccpredict.hgu.mrc.ac.uk/
MMRpro [33]	https://projects.iq.harvard.edu/bayesmendel/mmrpro
$PREMM_5$ [35]	http://premm.dfci.harvard.edu/

MMRpredict model was developed using colorectal cancer data from the patients and their relatives, and endometrial cancer data from their relatives [32]. MMRpro model was calculated using not only colorectal and endometrial cancers data but also microsatellite instability status [33]. PREMM model was revised two times, and current version is $PREMM_5$. The former version, $PREMM_{1,2,6}$, provided individual, gene-specific risk estimates for each of the three mismatch repair genes, such as *MLH1*, *MSH2*, and *MSH6* [36]; however, current version estimates the overall cumulative probability of having and *MLH1*, *MSH2*, *MSH6*, *PMS2*, and *EPCAM* gene mutation [35]. Green et al. investigated three prediction models (MMRpredict, MMRpro, and $PREMM_{1,2,6}$) for Lynch syndrome, and concluded that MMRpredict was the best-performing model for identifying colorectal cancer patients who are at high risk of Lynch syndrome [37]. However, the meta-analysis of these prediction models could not state that one model has a higher discrimination than any of the others, because of statistical variability, similar pooled area under curve values and the high degree of overlap in the confidence intervals [38]. Individuals with a quantified risk of 2.5% or greater on $PREMM_5$ or 5% or greater on MMRpro and MMRpredict are recommended for genetic evaluation referral and testing [35, 38, 39].

References

1. Win AK, Jenkins MA, Dowty JG, et al. Prevalence and penetrance of major genes and polygenes for colorectal cancer. Cancer Epidemiol Biomark Prev. 2017;26:404–12.
2. Vasen HF, Mecklin JP, Khan PM, Lynch HT. The International Collaborative Group on Hereditary Non-polyposis Colorectal Cancer (ICG-HNPCC). Dis Colon Rectum. 1991;34:424–5.
3. Bronner CE, Baker SM, Morrison PT, et al. Mutation in the DNA mismatch repair gene homolog hMLH1 is associated with hereditary nonpolyposis colorectal cancer. Nature. 1994;368:258–61.
4. Fishel R, Lescoe MK, Rao MR, et al. The human mutator gene homolog MSH2 and its association with hereditary nonpolyposis colorectal cancer. Cell. 1993;75:1027–38.
5. Miyaki M, Konishi M, Tanaka K, et al. Germline mutation of MSH6 as the cause of hereditary nonpolyposis colorectal cancer. Nat Genet. 1997;17:271–2.
6. Vasen HF, Watson P, Mecklin JP, Lynch HT. New clinical criteria for hereditary nonpolyposis colorectal cancer (HNPCC, Lynch syndrome) proposed by the International Collaborative group on HNPCC. Gastroenterology. 1999;116:1453–6.
7. Rodriguez-Bigas MA, Boland CR, Hamilton SR, et al. A National Cancer Institute Workshop on Hereditary Nonpolyposis Colorectal Cancer Syndrome: meeting highlights and Bethesda guidelines. J Natl Cancer Inst. 1997;89:1758–62.
8. Umar A, Boland CR, Terdiman JP, et al. Revised Bethesda guidelines for hereditary nonpolyposis colorectal cancer (Lynch syndrome) and microsatellite instability. J Natl Cancer Inst. 2004;96:261–8.

9. Moreira L, Balaguer F, Lindor N, et al. Identification of Lynch syndrome among patients with colorectal cancer. JAMA. 2012;308:1555–65.
10. Vasen HF. Clinical diagnosis and management of hereditary colorectal cancer syndromes. J Clin Oncol. 2000;18:81S–92.
11. Boland CR, Shike M. Report from the Jerusalem workshop on Lynch syndrome-hereditary nonpolyposis colorectal cancer. Gastroenterology. 2010;138:2197.e1–7.
12. Evaluation of Genomic Applications in Practice and Prevention (EGAPP) Working Group. Recommendations from the EGAPP Working Group: genetic testing strategies in newly diagnosed individuals with colorectal cancer aimed at reducing morbidity and mortality from Lynch syndrome in relatives. Genet Med. 2009;11:35–41.
13. Giardiello FM, Allen JI, Axilbund JE, et al. Guidelines on genetic evaluation and management of Lynch syndrome: a consensus statement by the US Multi-society Task Force on colorectal cancer. Am J Gastroenterol. 2014;109:1159–79.
14. Giardiello FM, Allen JI, Axilbund JE, et al. Guidelines on genetic evaluation and management of Lynch syndrome: a consensus statement by the US Multi-society Task Force on colorectal cancer. Gastroenterology. 2014;147:502–26.
15. Giardiello FM, Allen JI, Axilbund JE, et al. Guidelines on genetic evaluation and management of Lynch syndrome: a consensus statement by the US Multi-society Task Force on colorectal cancer. Dis Colon Rectum. 2014;57:1025–48.
16. Giardiello FM, Allen JI, Axilbund JE, et al. Guidelines on genetic evaluation and management of Lynch syndrome: a consensus statement by the US Multi-society Task Force on colorectal cancer. Gastrointest Endosc. 2014;80:197–220.
17. Lancaster JM, Powell CB, Chen LM, Richardson DL, SGO Clinical Practice Committee. Society of Gynecologic Oncology statement on risk assessment for inherited gynecologic cancer predispositions. Gynecol Oncol. 2015;136:3–7.
18. Committee on Practice Bulletins-Gynecology, Society of Gynecologic Oncology. ACOG practice bulletin no. 147: Lynch syndrome. Obstet Gynecol. 2014;124:1042–54.
19. Green RF, Ari M, Kolor K, et al. Evaluating the role of public health in implementation of genomics-related recommendations: a case study of hereditary cancers using the CDC Science Impact Framework. Genet Med. 2018;21(1):28–37.
20. Hampel H, Frankel WL, Martin E, et al. Screening for the Lynch syndrome (hereditary nonpolyposis colorectal cancer). N Engl J Med. 2005;352:1851–60.
21. Mvundura M, Grosse SD, Hampel H, Palomaki GE. The cost-effectiveness of genetic testing strategies for Lynch syndrome among newly diagnosed patients with colorectal cancer. Genet Med. 2010;12:93–104.
22. Grosse SD, Palomaki GE, Mvundura M, Hampel H. The cost-effectiveness of routine testing for Lynch syndrome in newly diagnosed patients with colorectal cancer in the United States: corrected estimates. Genet Med. 2015;17:510–1.
23. Boland CR, Thibodeau SN, Hamilton SR, et al. A National Cancer Institute workshop on microsatellite instability for cancer detection and familial predisposition: development of international criteria for the determination of microsatellite instability in colorectal cancer. Cancer Res. 1998;58:5248–57.
24. Suraweera N, Duval A, Reperant M, et al. Evaluation of tumor microsatellite instability using five quasimonomorphic mononucleotide repeats and pentaplex PCR. Gastroenterology. 2002;123:1804–11.
25. Buhard O, Cattaneo F, Wong YF, et al. Multipopulation analysis of polymorphisms in five mononucleotide repeats used to determine the microsatellite instability status of human tumors. J Clin Oncol. 2006;24:241–51.
26. Murphy KM, Zhang S, Geiger T, et al. Comparison of the microsatellite instability analysis system and the Bethesda panel for the determination of microsatellite instability in colorectal cancers. J Mol Diagn. 2006;8:305–11.
27. Patil DT, Bronner MP, Portier BP, et al. A five-marker panel in a multiplex PCR accurately detects microsatellite instability-high colorectal tumors without control DNA. Diagn Mol Pathol. 2012;21:127–33.

28. Dietmaier W, Wallinger S, Bocker T, et al. Diagnostic microsatellite instability: definition and correlation with mismatch repair protein expression. Cancer Res. 1997;57:4749–56.
29. Xicola RM, Llor X, Pons E, et al. Performance of different microsatellite marker panels for detection of mismatch repair-deficient colorectal tumors. J Natl Cancer Inst. 2007;99:244–52.
30. Hall G, Clarkson A, Shi A, et al. Immunohistochemistry for PMS2 and MSH6 alone can replace a four antibody panel for mismatch repair deficiency screening in colorectal adenocarcinoma. Pathology. 2010;42:409–13.
31. Hampel H, Frankel WL, Martin E, Arnold M, et al. Feasibility of screening for Lynch syndrome among patients with colorectal cancer. J Clin Oncol. 2008;26:5783–8.
32. Barnetson RA, Tenesa A, Farrington SM, Nicholl ID, Cetnarskyj R, Porteous ME, Campbell H, Dunlop MG. Identification and survival of carriers of mutations in DNA mismatch-repair genes in colon cancer. N Engl J Med. 2006;354:2751–63.
33. Chen S, Wang W, Lee S, Nafa K, Lee J, Romans K, Watson P, Gruber SB, Euhus D, Kinzler KW, Jass J, Gallinger S, Lindor NM, Casey G, Ellis N, Giardiello FM, Offit K, Parmigiani G, Colon Cancer Family Registry. Prediction of germline mutations and cancer risk in the Lynch syndrome. JAMA. 2006;296:1479–87.
34. Balmaña J, Stockwell DH, Steyerberg EW, Stoffel EM, Deffenbaugh AM, Reid JE, Ward B, Scholl T, Hendrickson B, Tazelaar J, Burbidge LA, Syngal S. Prediction of MLH1 and MSH2 mutations in Lynch syndrome. JAMA. 2006;296:1469–78.
35. Kastrinos F, Uno H, Ukaegbu C, et al. Development and validation of the PREMM(5) model for comprehensive risk assessment of Lynch syndrome. J Clin Oncol. 2017;35:2165–72.
36. Kastrinos F, Steyerberg EW, Mercado R, et al. The PREMM(1,2,6) model predicts risk of MLH1, MSH2, and MSH6 germline mutations based on cancer history. Gastroenterology. 2011;140:73–81.
37. Green RC, Parfrey PS, Woods MO, Younghusband HB. Prediction of Lynch syndrome in consecutive patients with colorectal cancer. J Natl Cancer Inst. 2009;101:331–40.
38. Win AK, Macinnis RJ, Dowty JG, Jenkins MA. Criteria and prediction models for mismatch repair gene mutations: a review. J Med Genet. 2013;50:785–93.
39. Kastrinos F, Ojha RP, Leenen C, et al. Comparison of prediction models for Lynch syndrome among individuals with colorectal cancer. J Natl Cancer Inst. 2015;108(2):djv308.

Surveillance Colonoscopy for Lynch Syndrome Affected Individuals

9

Takeshi Nakajima

Abstract

In individuals with Lynch syndrome, gastroenterologists and/or endoscopists should have responsibilities for the surveillance colonoscopy of metachronous colorectal cancer in the residual colon and/or rectum after surgery. The same responsibility applies to another Lynch syndrome-associated cancer, ex gastric cancer, and duodenal cancer, and also to surveillance of the relatives who have the same pathogenic variant of Lynch syndrome proband. In this paper, we introduce recent guidelines and reports from multicenter study in addition to an outline of the risk of gastrointestinal cancer in individuals with Lynch syndrome.

Keywords

Lynch syndrome · Surveillance · Colorectal adenoma · Colorectal cancer Colonoscopy · Gastrointestinal endoscopy

9.1 Introduction

In individuals with Lynch syndrome (LS), it has been shown that the risk of developing colorectal cancer (CRC) is high including those with metachronous CRC after surgery for their primary CRC and it is necessary of surveillance colonoscopy (CS) in their lifetime for early detection of CRC and removal of precancerous lesion "adenoma" [1, 2]. In 2000, Jarvien et al. reported the results of surveillance CS in a controlled trial over 15 years period [3]. In this study, the incidence of CRC and survival were compared in two cohorts of at-risk members of 22 LS family as follows, (1) surveillance CS at 3-year intervals was arranged for 133 LS

T. Nakajima (✉)
Cancer Institute Hospital, Clinical Genetics, Tokyo, Japan
e-mail: takeshi.nakajima@jfcr.or.jp

N. Tomita (ed.), *Lynch Syndrome*, https://doi.org/10.1007/978-981-15-6891-6_9

individuals, (2) 119 control LS individuals had no surveillance CS. As result, the study showed that surveillance CS at 3-year intervals prevents more than halves the risk of CRC and decreases overall mortality of CRC by about 65% in LS families. However, some other observational studies have confirmed the occurrence of advanced CRC during the surveillance CS at 2- or 3-year intervals and therefore recommended a 1-year interval of surveillance CS if possible [4, 5]. As for the start timing of surveillance CS, there are many reports to recommend LS individuals from 20 to 25 years old [6].

9.2 Introductions of the Guidelines for Recommended Colonoscopy Surveillance for Lynch Syndrome Individuals

9.2.1 North America

9.2.1.1 National Comprehensive Cancer Network (NCCN) Clinical Practice Guidelines

"Genetic/Familial High-Risk Assessment:Colorectal" has been published in the National Comprehensive Cancer Network (NCCN) Clinical Practice Guidelines in the USA [7]. According to the NCCN guidelines, the target individuals are classified into the following three categories according to the pathological variations of the genetic test results of mismatch repair (MMR) gene (*MLH1*, *MSH2*, *MSH6*, *PMS2*, and *EPCAM*) in the family, (1) positive for familial LS pathogenic variant, (2) individuals whose genetic test are not done, (3) negative for familial LS pathogenic variant. For (1) and (2) group individuals, surveillance CS should be performed at the age of 20–25 or if CRC was diagnosed under 25 in a family, 2–5 years from the youngest diagnosis age (Table 9.1). And recommends to begin at the earliest age of the diagnosed of CRC in the family member and recommend repeated CS in every 1–2 years. In the case of group (3), it is recommended that the surveillance CS are referred according to CRC guidelines for average-risk individuals. In the case of (2), the patients who meet the revised Bethesda Guidelines, which is a criterion for screening test for LS (see separate section), or who meet the Amsterdam criteria (see separate section), or who have a prediction of one of the models (MMRpro, PREMM5 or MMRpredict) has a 5% predictive risk of LS is included.

9.2.1.2 The United States Multi-society Task Force

The Multi-Society Task Force in the USA, in collaboration with invited experts, developed guidelines to assist health care providers with the appropriate provision of genetic testing and management of individuals at risk for and affected LS individuals [8–10]. In this guideline, surveillance CS for CRC is recommended in individuals at risk (first-degree relatives of those affected) or affected with LS every 1–2 years, beginning between ages 20–25 years or 2–5 years before the youngest age of diagnosis of CRC in the family if diagnosed before age 25 years.

Table 9.1 CS surveillance in Lynch syndrome individuals for colorectal cancer: recommendations and guidelines from various professional societies

Site	Recommendation for colonoscopy	
	Age (years)	Interval (years)
National Comprehensive Cancer Network (NCCN)	20–25	1–2
	2–5 years prior to the earliest colon cancer if it is diagnosed before age 25	
United States Multi-Society Task Force (AGA)	Every 1–2 years beginning at age 20–25 or 2–5 years younger than youngest age at diagnosis of CRC in family if diagnosis before age 25	Annual colonoscopy in pathogenic MMR variant individuals
	MSH6: 30 *PMS2*/35	
American College of Gastroenterology (ACG)	20–25 (*MLH1/MSH2* pathogenic variant)	1–2
	25–30 (*MSH6/PMS2* pathogenic variant)	
American Society of Clinical Oncology (ASCO)	Starting at age 20–25	1–2 (No upper limit is established.)
	5 years before the youngest case in the family	
European Society for Medical Oncology (ESMO)	*MLH1/MSH2*:25	1–2
	MSH6/PMS2:35	
European Hereditary Tumour Group (formerly the Malloca Group)	20–25	1–2
European Society of Digestive Oncology	20–25 (Chromoendoscopy)	1–2
Guidelines for the management of hereditary colorectal cancer from the British Society of Gastroenterology (BSG)/Association of Coloproctology of Great Britain and Ireland (ACPGBI)/ United Kingdom Cancer Genetics Group (UKCGG)	*MLH1/MSH2*:25	2 yearly until age 75 years
	MSH6/PMS2:35	2 yearly until age 75 years

9.2.1.3 American College of Gastroenterology

American College of Gastroenterology (ACG) also has reported recommendations as follows, in individuals at risk for or affected with LS, surveillance CS should be performed at least every 2 years, beginning between ages 20 and 25 years. Annual surveillance CS should be considered in the case with pathogenic variant in MMR gene [11].

9.2.1.4 American Society of Clinical Oncology

American Society of Clinical Oncology (ASCO) also reported their guidelines in 2015 [12]. The possibility of a hereditary cancer syndrome should be assessed for each patient at the time of CRC diagnosis. In LS individuals, surveillance CS every 1–2 years, should be started at age 20–25 or 5 years before the youngest case in the family. No upper limit should be established for surveillance CS.

9.2.2 Guidelines in European Countries

9.2.2.1 European Society for Medical Oncology (ESMO) Guidelines

In 2019, ESMO guidelines committee has also showed the recommended method of surveillance CS [13]. Since the diagnosis of CRC before age 25 is unlikely in individuals with LS, and the CRC risk in person with *MSH6* and *PMS2* pathogenic variant is substantially lower than those with *MLH1* or *MSH2* pathogenic variant, starting timing of surveillance CS is recommended at the age of 25 years for LS individuals with *MLH1* or *MSH2* pathogenic variant and at the age of 35 years for LS individuals with *MSH6* or *PMS2* pathogenic variant. In all cases, age of onset in the youngest member of the family is to be considered and surveillance CS should be started 5 years earlier. Surveillance CS every 1–2 years in asymptomatic LS individuals is recommended.

9.2.2.2 European Hereditary Tumor Group (Formerly the Malloca Group) Guideline

In 2007, a group of European experts (the Mallorca group) published guidelines for the clinical management of LS [14]. Since then substantial new information has become available necessitating an update of the guidelines. In 2011 and 2012 workshops were organized in Palma de Mallorca. A 3-year interval between colonoscopies has been proved to be effective. In view of the observation of (advanced) CRC detected between 2 and 3 years after surveillance CS, the recommended interval for pathogenic variant individuals is 1–2 years [6].

9.2.2.3 European Society of Digestive Oncology

In 2018, the objective of the European Society of Digestive Oncology (ESDO) expert discussion 2018 at the 20th World Congress on Gastrointestinal Cancer was to review the current approach to individuals and individuals at risk for the aforementioned hereditary GI cancers [15]. Individuals diagnosed with a pathogenic germline variant in any MMR gene should undergo surveillance CS at least every 1–2 years, as surveillance CS is the only means to reduce mortality. Whenever possible, surveillance CS should be performed as chromoendoscopy using indigo carmine.

9.2.2.4 British Society of Gastroenterology (BSG)/Association of Coloproctology of Great Britain and Ireland (ACPGBI)/ United Kingdom Cancer Genetics Group (UKCGG)

This guideline is an update from the 2010 British Society of Gastroenterology/ Association of Coloproctology of Great Britain and Ireland (BSG/ACPGBI) guidelines for surveillance CS in moderate and high-risk groups [16]. It recommends that surveillance CS should be performed at a 2-year interval for all LS individuals. Surveillance CS is recommended from age 25 years for *MLH1* and *MSH2* pathogenic variant individuals and 35 years for *MSH6* and *PMS2* pathogenic variant individuals.

9.3 Resent Report of Colorectal Cancer Surveillance in Lynch Syndrome Individuals

Recently, several prospective cohorts study group for LS have been established in Europe and the USA, one of which is "The Prospective Lynch Syndrome Database (PLSD)" of the European Hereditary Tumor Group (EHTG) [17]. In the beginning of this enrollment, total number of 1942 LS individuals without cancer were already registered [18]. Follow-up of cancer-free individuals with pathogenic MMR variants in any of the *MLH1*, *MSH2*, *MSH6*, and *PMS2* genes showed a cumulative incidence of CRC cancer at age 70 years of 46%, 35%, 20%, and 10%, respectively. The effectiveness of continuous surveillance CS has been proven. When browsing the PLSD homepage, online software is available that displays a graph of morbidity risk for LS-related cancers by gender, cancer history, and affected gene. It is a quite useful tool to demonstrate the LS-associated cancer risk to LS individuals in genetic counseling.

Next, in 2018, additional analysis results of 3119 individuals including cancer patients were reported [19]. Cumulative CRC incidence at age 75 years in LS for pathological variants of *MLH1*, *MSH2*, *and MSH6* was 46%, 43%, and 15%. In all of the above data, cancer risk was reported 0 in LS patients with *PMS2* pathogenic variant, but Broeke et al. reported the CRC risk in LS individuals with *PMS2* pathogenic variant [20]. Segregation analysis of *PMS2* pathogenic variants in all 284 families (4878 first- and second-degree relatives) showed the incidence of CRC cancer as 13% [95% CI, 7.9–22%] for man and 12% for women [95% CI, 6.7–21%]. The risk of LS-associated cancers other than the large intestine is not so high, and only surveillance CS may be enough.

In 2018, Engel et al. reported comparisons the results of surveillance CS for LS individuals performed in Germany, the Netherlands, and Finland [21]. The recommended CS intervals in the three countries are different as every year, every 1–2 years, and every 2–3 years, respectively. However, as a result, CRC incidence and stage classification at the time of detection were reported to be not significantly different between the three countries. In this comparison study, from 1984 to 2015, 16,327 surveillance CSs were performed for 2747 LS individuals (*MLH1*, *MSH2*, *MSH6*), and they were classified into two groups based on the presence or absence of CRC at the time of the first CS. The cumulative incidence of CRC at 10 years ranged from 4.1 to 18.4%. In the group without a past history of CRC, the incidence of adenoma was higher in Germany compared to other countries, but other results did not differ in the incidence of adenoma or CRC. Despite the short examination interval, the incidence of CRC was relatively high. Contrary to their initial expectations, they did not detect an association of shorter intervals with a lower incidence of CRC. They discussed that there are some possible hypothesis for this finding. In sporadic CRC, it is generally agreed that the development of CRC from adenomas takes 10 years or more. In LS individuals, however, small adenomas may develop and convert to CRC much faster, perhaps even within 1–2 years. As a consequence, the time window for the detection of adenomas might be so short that most adenomas become malignant before detection, even with annual CS. The true purpose of surveillance CS is not only to control CRC mortality but also to control CRC morbidity and to reduce surgical resection. Physicians need to understand the carcinogenesis of CRC in LS individuals and then should perform high-quality surveillance CSs. For limitation of this study, only adenoma detection rate, but no other data (bowel preparation status, cecal intubation rate, observation time) on the quality of individual colonoscopies, was available.

9.4 Molecular Pathway of Colorectal Cancer Carcinogenesis in Lynch Syndrome

It is important for physician who performs surveillance CS to understand the carcinogenesis of CRC in LS individuals. Colorectal adenomas with LS individuals may be young onset (<40 years) and present with MSI-H. Even if smaller than sporadic adenomas, they may be more atypical phenotype and have a shorter time to cancer [22, 23]. Kloor et al. systematically analyzed non-tumorous colon mucosa from 10 LS patients and control non-LS patients ($N = 9$) for MMR protein expression (*MLH1*, *MSH2*, and *EPCAM*) with immunohistochemistry [24]. They reported the existence of MMR-deficient foci in normally appearance colon mucosa only in LS patient. Tanaka et al. reported that MMR deficiency was more frequent in adenomas obtained from older patients (aged ≥60 years; 81 of 86, 94%), with larger tumor size (>5 mm; 71 of 73, 97%) and with high-grade dysplasia (50 of 51, 98%) [25]. Recently, Ahadova et al. reported three molecular pathways model of carcinogenesis CRC in LS individuals [26]. They had evaluated the frequency of MMR deficiency by immunohistochemistry in adenomas from LS individuals. Some CRCs were found to grow from MMR-proficient adenomas after secondary inactivation of the MMR system. However, most CRCs developed from MMR-deficient precursor lesions, either via an adenomatous phase or as non-polyposis lesions. Therefore, endoscopists need to find and resect not only polypoid-type but also non-polypoid-type precancerous colorectal lesions during surveillance CS. Colonoscopists might perform aggressive endoscopic resection regardless of size when detecting neoplastic lesion during surveillance CS. And if MMR deficiency is present in resected polyps in normal patients, especially for adenomas greater than 5 mm and/or high-grade dysplasia, genetic counseling should be conducted to consider genetic testing for MMR gene.

9.5 Colonoscopy Quality Assurance

In the aforementioned prospective cohort studies in western countries, colorectal neoplasia was discovered during surveillance CS including not only adenoma and intramucosal cancers but also many advanced cancers. Since the true end point of surveillance CS in LS individuals is the suppression of the development of advanced cancer, this result needs to be further investigated. When performing CS and examining its effects, it is necessary to guarantee the quality of the CS. These reports lack the description about bowel preparation status, cecal intubation rate, observation time, adenoma detection rate, polyp detection rate, etc., indicating the degree of quality control of CS.

Ramhi et al. conducted a prospective, multicenter, randomized trial to compare standard CS with standard CS followed by pancolonicchromoscopy with indigo carmine in LS individuals [27]. A total of 78 eligible patients (median age, 45 years) were enrolled at ten centers from July 2008 to August 2009. Significantly more patients with at least one adenoma were identified by chromocolonoscopy (32/78 (41%)) than by standard CS (18/78 (23%); $P < 0.001$). The results support the proposition that chromocolonoscopy may significantly improve the detection rate of colorectal adenomas in patients undergoing surveillance CS for LS individuals.

In French clinical groups, quality control of CS was tried to be achieved in LS individuals, resulting in a reduction in CRC detection rate to 1/353 (0.3%) [28]. Starting at the age of 20, CS with blue indigo carmine was scheduled every 2 years. In cases of incomplete CS, insufficient bowel preparation, absence of chromoendoscopy achievement or adenoma detection, the interval between surveillance CS was adjusted. The optimal preparation was defined with a sufficient bowel preparation according to endoscopist appreciation or defined as a Boston scale >6 with an underscore per segment >2. And if adenoma was detected in the exam, the next exam is proposed within 1 year (±3 months). This French protocol should be refereed in also large prospective studies.

9.6 The Usefulness of Image Enhanced Colonoscopy

In addition to white light observation, studies on the usefulness of advanced imaging modalities [autofluorescence, flexible spectal imaging, and narrowband imaging (NBI)] have also been reported. First, East et al. reported the usefulness of NBI [29]. 62 patients from hereditary non-polyposis colorectal cancer (HNPCC) families (Amsterdam II or genetic criteria) attending for surveillance CS were examined twice from cecum to sigmoid–descending junction, first with high-definition white light and then a second pass with NBI in a back-to-back fashion. At least one adenoma in the proximal colon was detected during the initial white light pass in 17/62 (27%). NBI detected additional adenomas in 17/62 (27%). They concluded that use of NBI in the proximal colon for LS patients undergoing surveillance CS appears to improve adenoma detection, particularly those with a flat morphology.

Cellier et al. conducted a prospective multicenter trial in a back-to-back fashion to compare the third-generation NBI with surveillance CS with indigo carmine chromoendoscopy (ICC) for detecting colonic adenomas in LS patients [30]. 138 patients underwent a double CS, first with NBI, followed by ICC, in a back-to-back design. At least one adenoma was detected during the initial NBI CS in 28 patients

(20.3%), and 42 patients (30.4%) had at least one adenoma detected after both NBI and ICC (difference, 10.1%; 95% confidence interval, −0.1–20.3%).

Rivero-Sánchez et al. conducted a parallel controlled study, from July 2016 through January 2018 at 14 centers in Spain of adults with pathogenic germline variants in mismatch repair genes (60% women; mean age, 47 ± 14 years) under surveillance CS [31]. They found an important overlap of confidence intervals (CIs) and no significant difference in adenoma detection rates by pancolonic chromoendoscopy (34.4%; 95% CI 26.4–43.3%) versus white light endoscopy (28.1%; 95% CI 21.1–36.4%; $P = 0.28$). In conclusion they found that surveillance CS for LS individuals, high-definition white light endoscopy is not inferior to pancolonic chromoendoscopy if performed by experienced and dedicated endoscopists in this randomized parallel trial.

For standard surveillance CS, to improve visualization and reduce the blind spot of colonic mucosa and to increase adenoma detection rate (ADR) and polyp detection rate (PDR), many endoscopic techniques and technologies have been developed. Moriyama et al. reviewed about the advanced technology of CS, such as the Third Eye Retroscope (TER; Avantis Medical Systems, Sunnyvale, CA, USA), FULL Spectrum Endoscopy System colonoscope (FUSE; EndoChoice, Alpharetta, GA, USA), extra-wide-angle-view colonoscope (OLYMPUS, Tokyo, Japan), which were seem to be promising for improving ADR and PDR [32]. Castaneda et al. conducted a systematic review to compare the ADR, polyp detection rate (PDR), and adenoma miss rate (AMR) between new technology devices (NTDs) and conventional CS and between mechanical and optical NTDs. They divided NTDs into two groups based on their mechanism of action: mechanical NTDs [Endocuff (Arc Medical, Leeds, UK), G-Eye (SMART Medical Systems Ltd., Ra'anana, Israel), and Endorings (EndoAid Ltd., Caesarea, Israel)] and optical NTDs [Third Eye (Avantis Medical Systems Inc., Sunnyvale, Calif) and full-spectrum CS (FUSE; EndoChoice, Alpharetta, Ga)] [33]. They concluded that NTDs are an effective option to improve ADR and PDR and decrease AMR, particularly with mechanical NTDs. For surveillance CS study for LS, these NTSs would be beneficial not to miss precursor lesions of CRCs.

References

1. Rex DK, Kahi CJ, Levin B, et al. Guidelines for colonoscopy surveillance after cancer resection: a consensus update by the American Cancer Society and the US Multi-Society Task Force on Colorectal Cancer. Gastroenterology. 2006;130(6):1865–71.
2. Mecklin JP, Aarnio M, Laara E, et al. Development of colorectal tumors in colonoscopic surveillance in Lynch syndrome. Gastroenterology. 2007;133(4):1093–8.
3. Jarvinen HJ, Aarnio M, Mustonen H, et al. Controlled 15-year trial on screening for colorectal cancer in families with hereditary nonpolyposis colorectal cancer. Gastroenterology. 2000;118(5):829–34.
4. Vasen HF, Nagengast FM, Khan PM. Interval cancers in hereditary non-polyposis colorectal cancer (Lynch syndrome). Lancet. 1995;345(8958):1183–4.
5. Engel C, Rahner N, Schulmann K, et al. Efficacy of annual colonoscopic surveillance in individuals with hereditary nonpolyposis colorectal cancer. Clin Gastroenterol Hepatol. 2010;8(2):174–82.

6. Vasen HF, Blanco I, Aktan-Collan K, et al. Revised guidelines for the clinical management of Lynch syndrome (HNPCC): recommendations by a group of European experts. Gut. 2013;62(6):812–23.
7. National Comprehensive Cancer Network. NCCN guidelines: genetic/familial high-risk assessment: colorectal (Version I. 2018-July 12, 2018). Accessed 1 Apr 2018.
8. Giardiello FM, Allen JI, Axilbund JE, et al. Guidelines on genetic evaluation and management of Lynch syndrome: a consensus statement by the US Multi-society Task Force on colorectal cancer. Am J Gastroenterol. 2014;109(8):1159–79.
9. Giardiello FM, Allen JI, Axilbund JE, et al. Guidelines on genetic evaluation and management of Lynch syndrome: a consensus statement by the US Multi-Society Task Force on colorectal cancer. Gastroenterology. 2014;147(2):502–26.
10. Giardiello FM, Allen JI, Axilbund JE, et al. Guidelines on genetic evaluation and management of Lynch syndrome: a consensus statement by the US Multi-Society Task Force on Colorectal Cancer. Dis Colon Rectum. 2014;57(8):1025–48.
11. Syngal S, Brand RE, Church JM, et al. ACG clinical guideline: genetic testing and management of hereditary gastrointestinal cancer syndromes. Am J Gastroenterol. 2015;110(2):223–62. quiz 263
12. Stoffel EM, Mangu PB, Gruber SB, et al. Hereditary colorectal cancer syndromes: American Society of Clinical Oncology Clinical Practice Guideline endorsement of the familial risk-colorectal cancer: European Society for Medical Oncology Clinical Practice Guidelines. J Clin Oncol. 2015;33(2):209–17.
13. Stjepanovic N, Moreira L, Carneiro F, et al. Hereditary gastrointestinal cancers: ESMO Clinical Practice Guidelines for diagnosis, treatment and follow-updagger. Ann Oncol. 2019;30(10):1558–71.
14. Vasen HF, Moslein G, Alonso A, et al. Guidelines for the clinical management of Lynch syndrome (hereditary non-polyposis cancer). J Med Genet. 2007;44(6):353–62.
15. Vangala DB, Cauchin E, Balmana J, et al. Screening and surveillance in hereditary gastrointestinal cancers: recommendations from the European Society of Digestive Oncology (ESDO) expert discussion at the 20th European Society for Medical Oncology (ESMO)/World Congress on Gastrointestinal Cancer, Barcelona, June 2018. Eur J Cancer. 2018;104:91–103.
16. Monahan KJ, Bradshaw N, Dolwani S, et al. Guidelines for the management of hereditary colorectal cancer from the British Society of Gastroenterology (BSG)/Association of Coloproctology of Great Britain and Ireland (ACPGBI)/United Kingdom Cancer Genetics Group (UKCGG). Gut. 2020;69(3):411–44.
17. Prospective Lynch Syndrome Database (PLSD)—cumulative risk for cancer by age, genetic variant, and gender. https://ehtg.org/collaborative-studies/plsd/
18. Moller P, Seppala T, Bernstein I, et al. Cancer incidence and survival in Lynch syndrome patients receiving colonoscopic and gynaecological surveillance: first report from the prospective Lynch syndrome database. Gut. 2017;66(3):464–72.
19. Moller P, Seppala TT, Bernstein I, et al. Cancer risk and survival in path_MMR carriers by gene and gender up to 75 years of age: a report from the Prospective Lynch Syndrome Database. Gut. 2018;67(7):1306–16.
20. Ten Broeke SW, van der Klift HM, Tops CMJ, et al. Cancer risks for PMS2-associated Lynch syndrome. J Clin Oncol. 2018;36(29):2961–8.
21. Engel C, Vasen HF, Seppala T, et al. No difference in colorectal Cancer incidence or stage at detection by colonoscopy among 3 countries with different Lynch syndrome surveillance policies. Gastroenterology. 2018;155(5):1400–9. e1402
22. Jass JR, Stewart SM. Evolution of hereditary non-polyposis colorectal cancer. Gut. 1992;33(6):783–6.
23. Jass JR, Cottier DS, Pokos V, Parry S, Winship IM. Mixed epithelial polyps in association with hereditary non-polyposis colorectal cancer providing an alternative pathway of cancer histogenesis. Pathology. 1997;29(1):28–33.
24. Kloor M, Huth C, Voigt AY, et al. Prevalence of mismatch repair-deficient crypt foci in Lynch syndrome: a pathological study. Lancet Oncol. 2012;13(6):598–606.

25. Tanaka M, Nakajima T, Sugano K, et al. Mismatch repair deficiency in Lynch syndrome-associated colorectal adenomas is more prevalent in older patients. Histopathology. 2016;69(2):322–8.
26. Ahadova A, Gallon R, Gebert J, et al. Three molecular pathways model colorectal carcinogenesis in Lynch syndrome. Int J Cancer. 2018;143(1):139–50.
27. Rahmi G, Lecomte T, Malka D, et al. Impact of chromoscopy on adenoma detection in patients with Lynch syndrome: a prospective, multicenter, blinded, tandem colonoscopy study. Am J Gastroenterol. 2015;110(2):288–98.
28. Perrod G, Samaha E, Rahmi G, et al. Impact of an optimized colonoscopic screening program for patients with Lynch syndrome: 6-year results of a specialized French network. Ther Adv Gastroenterol. 2018;11:1756284818775058.
29. East JE, Suzuki N, Stavrinidis M, Guenther T, Thomas HJ, Saunders BP. Narrow band imaging for colonoscopic surveillance in hereditary non-polyposis colorectal cancer. Gut. 2008;57(1):65–70.
30. Cellier C, Perrod G, Colas C, et al. Back-to-back comparison of colonoscopy with virtual chromoendoscopy using a third-generation narrow-band imaging system to chromoendoscopy with indigo carmine in patients with Lynch syndrome. Am J Gastroenterol. 2019;114(10):1665–70.
31. Rivero-Sanchez L, Arnau-Collell C, Herrero J, et al. White-light endoscopy is adequate for Lynch syndrome surveillance in a randomized and noninferiority study. Gastroenterology. 2020;158(4):895–904. e891
32. Moriyama T, Uraoka T, Esaki M, Matsumoto T. Advanced technology for the improvement of adenoma and polyp detection during colonoscopy. Dig Endosc. 2015;27(Suppl 1):40–4.
33. Castaneda D, Popov VB, Verheyen E, Wander P, Gross SA. New technologies improve adenoma detection rate, adenoma miss rate, and polyp detection rate: a systematic review and meta-analysis. Gastrointest Endosc. 2018;88(2):209–222.e211.

10 Surgical Approach for Colorectal Cancer in Patients with Lynch Syndrome

Hideyuki Ishida, Keiichiro Ishibashi, and Kensuke Kumamoto

Abstract

Lynch syndrome (LS) is caused by pathogenic variants of one of DNA mismatch repair genes (*MLH1*, *MSH2*, *MSH6*, *PMS2*) or 3′ deletion of *EPCAM* in the germline. Colorectal cancer (CRC) is a hallmark of the syndrome, and the cumulative risk of CRC ranges from 10 to 46% by 70 years old, depending on the gene affected. Moreover, despite the high cumulative risk of subsequent CRC (metachronous CRC) after the first CRC is managed with surgery, the optimal surgical treatment is controversial. Prophylactic colorectal resection prior to CRC development is not recommended regardless of the type of surgery. Recent studies and our analysis show that the risk of metachronous CRC is considerably higher following segmental colectomy as compared to extended colectomy among patients with genetically proven LS. However, overall survival did not differ between patients with two different surgical procedures. The choice of surgical procedures for the first rectal cancer is complicated because of insufficient data available and thus needs further investigations. Surgical procedures for first CRC in patients with LS may depend on various factors that may vary among individuals, including the timing of genetic diagnosis (before or after the first CRC development), age at CRC diagnosis, site of CRC, genes affected, and expected quality of life. Individuals with genetically proven LS must be counselled prior to any surgical intervention for first CRC. In summary, an extended colectomy may be currently the most effective surgical technique to reduce the risk of metachronous colon cancer.

H. Ishida (✉) · K. Ishibashi
Department of Digestive Tract and General Surgery, Saitama Medical Center, Saitama Medical University, Kawagoe, Saitama, Japan
e-mail: 05hishi@saitama-med.ac.jp

K. Kumamoto
Department of Gastroenterological Surgery, Faculty of Medicine, Kagawa University, Kita-gun, Kagawa, Japan

N. Tomita (ed.), *Lynch Syndrome*, https://doi.org/10.1007/978-981-15-6891-6_10

Keywords

Lynch syndrome · Colorectal surgery · Colectomy · Proctocolectomy Metachronous colorectal cancer

10.1 Introduction

Colorectal cancer (CRC) is the fourth most frequently diagnosed malignancy and the second leading cause of cancer-related death globally [1]. Lynch syndrome (LS) is an autosomal dominant condition caused by pathogenic variants in one of DNA mismatch repair (MMR) genes (*MLH1*, *MSH2*, *MSH6*, and *PMS2*) or 3′ deletion of *EPCAM* in the germline line [2]. Carriers of the LS pathogenic variant are at increased risk for various cancers at a young age including CRC and endometrial cancer. The European "Mallorca group" and the International Society for Gastrointestinal Hereditary Tumours recently reported that the lifetime risk of CRC by age 70 years is approximately 10–46%, depending on the gene affected [3, 4]. LS-associated CRC is characterized by right-sided predominance, low incidence in the rectum, and high incidence of synchronous and metachronous occurrence [2, 5]. These characteristics might influence the choice of surgical procedures, the timing of genetic diagnosis (before or after surgical interventions), and long-term quality of life that is potentially altered by different surgical procedures.

Segmental colectomy (SC), which comprises right hemicolectomy, left colectomy, sigmoid colectomy, or other segmental resection of the colon segment, is a standard surgical procedure for LS-associated CRC regardless of the timing of genetic diagnosis. Considering the increased risk of metachronous CRC in individuals with genetically proven LS that develop CRC, more extended colectomy (EC), which comprises subtotal colectomy with ileosigmoidal anastomosis or total colectomy with ileorectal anastomosis, should be considered for the first CRC. The optimal surgical approach for CRC patients with LS remains unclear to date because of the lack of randomized controlled trials comparing SC and EC. In addition, the oncological outcomes of LS patients with rectal cancer diagnosed with first CRC have not been well-examined because of its low prevalence. In this chapter, we reviewed the surgical approaches and outcomes in patients with genetically proven LS who underwent surgical resection for first CRC to guide decision-making for the optimal surgical approach in these patients.

10.2 Baseline Characteristics of LS-Associated CRC Updated

Baseline characteristics of LS-associated CRC have been previously reported; however, the majority of previous studies enrolled patients who fulfilled clinical criteria such as the revised Amsterdam criteria and/or those characterized with high penetrance of CRC, that is, those with proven pathogenic variant in *MLH1* or *MSH2*.

Recent advances in genetic diagnosis of LS and the widespread use of universal LS-associated tumor screening have led to the updating of characteristics of LS-associated CRC, which is an important factor in surgical treatment.

The "Mallorca group" [3] has recently conducted a prospective study of 1942 individuals with germline pathogenic variants of *MLH1*, *MSH2*, *MSH6*, and *PMS2* and reported the revised estimates of the different penetrance of CRC. These 1942 individuals who did not develop previously cancer had colonoscopic surveillance for a total of 13782 observation years. Among those with first cancer, the cumulative incidences of CRC at 70 years by gene were 46%, 35%, 20%, and 10% for *MLH1*, *MSH2*, *MSH6*, and *PMS2* carriers, respectively.

Kim et al. [5] reported the tumor location of first CRC and synchronous CRC in 114 LS patients with a mean age of 43 years (range, 24–82 years) who were referred to genetic testing through universal tumor screening. The tumor was located in the right colon, left colon, and the rectum in 74 (69.8%), 21 (19.8%), and 11 (10.4%) patients. Synchronous CRC developed in 12 (11.3%), while metachronous CRC developed in 13 (11.4%). Approximately half (54%) of the metachronous CRCs were located in the right colon, while four (31%) were in the rectum.

Hiatt et al. [6] analyzed 64 LS patients who underwent SC for proximal colon cancer and reported that 6 (46%) of the 13 patients who developed metachronous CRC, developed it again in the remaining proximal colon.

Win et al. [7] analyzed 79 LS patients with first rectal cancer treated with abdominal perineal resection or anterior resection and reported that 21 metachronous CRCs developed, 16 (76%) of which were in the proximal colon (cecum, ascending colon, hepatic flexure, or transverse colon).

10.3 Surgical Treatment for CRC in LS

10.3.1 Prophylactic Surgery

In the past, prophylactic colorectal resection such as total proctocolectomy with ileorectal anastomosis or total proctocolectomy with ileal pouch-anal anastomosis (IPAA) prior to first CRC development was performed in selected individuals with LS or hereditary nonpolyposis CRC (HNPCC) [8] without genetic diagnosis. However, because of the lower penetrance of CRC in carriers of the LS pathogenic variant than patients with familial adenomatous polyposis, prophylactic colorectal resection should not be performed regardless of the type of resection.

10.3.2 Metachronous Risk of CRC Following SC vs. EC for First Colon Cancer

Heneghan et al. [9], Anele et al. [10], and Malik et al. [11] conducted systematic reviews and meta-analyses to investigate the risk of metachronous CRC following SC for first CRC compared to EC (Table 10.1). Of these studies, Malik et al. [11]

Table 10.1 Systematic reviews and meta-analyses investigating the risk of metachnonous colorectal cancer (CRC) following segmental colectomy (SC) compared to extended colectomy (EC)

Author	Year	Year of publication of studies retrieved	Number of studies retrieved	Number of cases (SC/EC)	Metachronous CRC (SC vs. EC)	Overall survival (SC vs. EC)	Genetic testing for mismatch repair genes
Heneghan et al.	2015	1993–2012	6	948 (780/168)	23.5% vs. 6.8% (OR: 3.69, 95% CI: 1.889–7.125, $P < 0.005$)	10-year: 90.7% vs. 89.7% (OR: 1.92, 95% CI: 0.915–4.035, $P = 0.09$)	Four of six studies included genetically proven LS
Anele et al.	2017	2002–2015	6	871 (705/166)	22.6% vs. 6.0% (OR: 4.02, 95% CI: 2.01–8.04, $P < 0.001$)	Not documented	Six studies included genetically proven LS
Malik et al.	2018	1993–2017	10	1389 (1119/270)	Genetically proven LS: OR: 8.56, 95% CI: 3.37–21.73, $P < 0.01$; Meeting Amsterdam criteria only: OR: 3.04; 95% CI: 1.46–6.34, $P < 0.01$	OR: 1.65, 95% CI: 0.90–3.02	Six of ten studies included genetically proven LS. Meeting Amsterdam criteria only ($n = 508$), Genetically proven LS ($n = 881$)

OR Odds ratio, *CI* confidence interval, *LS* Lynch syndrome evaluated the largest cases and reported the genetically proven cases separately from those who were not. They demonstrated that among patients with genetically proven, the risk of metachronous CRC development was 8.56-fold higher following SC as compared with EC. Similarly, the risk was also higher (3.04-fold) following SC among patients meeting the Amsterdam criteria only. This result seems reasonable because the cohort comprised patients meeting the Amsterdam criteria, which potentially included patients with familial CRC type X [12] who are known to have a lower risk of metachronous CRC than LS patients. The risk of metachronous CRC following SC as compared with EC reported by Heneghan et al. [9] and Anele et al. [10] seems to concur with that reported by Malik et al. [11].

However, the findings of these studies should be interpreted with caution as they included a significant proportion of patients with first rectal cancer who were regarded to have undergone "colectomy." In addition, these studies included both patients with genetically proven LS and those who fulfilled the Amsterdam criteria only. Despite the useful information they provided, these three systematic reviews and meta-analyses contain inappropriate studies to strictly evaluate the optimal surgical procedures for patients with CRC in LS. Specifically, the study by Natarajan et al. [13], which was included in all the three systematic reviews and meta-analyses, included patients who underwent EC prior to the development of first CRC as a prophylactic treatment. In the study by Win et al. [7], which was included in the systematic review and meta-analysis by Malik et al. [11], all the patients had rectal cancer and were classified into segmental resection group only.

We retrieved five studies comparing SC and EC among patients with genetically proven LS only that were reported between January 2011 and September 2018 (Table 10.2). Similar with findings in previous studies, metachronous CRC was found to occur more frequently in patients who underwent SC (144/639, 22.5%) than in patients who underwent EC (7/215, 3.3%) during long-term follow-up. Collectively, these findings indicate that compared with SC, EC can reduce metachronous CRC in LS patients with first colon cancer. However, we should note that there may be substantial selection bias because patients selected for EC were more likely to have been genetically diagnosed with LS preoperatively and were likely to have stage I cancer than those who underwent SC.

10.3.3 Risk Factors for Metachronous CRC Following SC for First Colon Cancer

Identifying the risk factors for metachronous CRC following SC for first colon (CRC) cancer is important because most patients with LS-associated CRC underwent genetic diagnosis for MMR deficiency following SC for first CRC. The risk factors for metachronous CRC after SC have been reported previously. Kim et al. [5] reported that bowel resection ≥25 cm decreased the risk compared with less extensive resection (hazard ratio (HR): 0.10; 95% confidence interval (CI): 0.01–0.86). Parry et al. [14] also reported that the risk of metachronous CRC significantly reduced by 31% (95% CI: 12–46%, $P = 0.002$) for every 10 cm of bowel

Table 10.2 Recent publications (2011–2018) comparing between segmental colectomy and extended colectomy in colorectal cancer (CRC) patients with genetically confirmed Lynch syndrome

Author	Year	Country	Study design	Number of patients	Affected genes	Tumor location	Segmental resection/ Extended resection	Frequency of metachronous CRC (segmental resection vs. extended resection)	Cumulative risk of metachronous CRC (segmental resection vs. extended resection)	Disease-specific (DS) or CRC-specific[a] survival rate (segmental resection vs. extended resection)	Overall survival rate (segmental resection vs. extended resection)
Parry et al.[a]	2011	USA, Canada, Australia, New Zealand	Retrospective	382	*MLH1* ($n = 172$), *MSH2* ($n = 167$), *MSH6* ($n = 23$), *PMS2* ($n = 20$)	Right colon ($n = 241$), left colon ($n = 73$), rectosigmoid ($n = 14$), unknown ($n = 4$)	332/50	74 (22.3%) vs. 0 (0%)	16 % at 10 years and 41% at 20 years vs. 0% at 10 and 20 years (*P*-value not documented	Not documented	Not documented
Stupart et al.	2011	South Africa	Prospective	60	*MLH1* ($n = 42$), *MSH2* ($n = 18$)	Colon only ($n = 60$)	39/21	8 (20.5%) vs. 2 (9.5%)	41% vs. 0% at 15 years (*P*-value not documented)	Survival rates not specifically documented ($P = 0.048$, in favor of patients with extended resection), CRC-specific survial	Survival rates not specifically documented ($P = 0.29$)
Kim et al.	2017	Republic of Korea	Retrospective	106	*MLH1*($n = 64$), *MSH2* ($n = 27$), *MSH6* ($n = 4$), *EPCAM* ($n = 11$)	Right colon ($n = 74$), left colon ($n = 21$), rectum ($n = 11$)	76/30	13 (17.1%) vs. 0 (0%)	20.4% vs. 0% at 10 years ($P = 0.04$)	Survival rates not specifically documented ($P = 0.66$)[a], CRC-specific survival	83.3% vs. 82.9% at 15 years ($P = 0.28$)

Renkonen-Sinisalo et al.	2017	Finland	Retrospective	242	*MLH1* ($n = 98$), *MSH2* ($n = 36$), *MSH6* ($n = 8$)	Colon only ($n = 242$)	144/98	36 (25%) vs. 5 (5%)	46.6% vs. 9.6% at 25 years ($P < 0.001$)	82.7% vs. 87.2% in 25 years ($P = 0.76$), DS survival	Survival rates not specifically documented ($P = 0.83$)
Hiatt et al.	2018	USA	Retrospective	64	*MLH1* ($n = 39$), *MSH2* ($n = 20$), *MSH6* ($n = 1$), *EPCAM* ($n = 2$), >1 mutation ($n = 2$)	Right colon only ($n = 64$)	48/16	13 (27%) vs. 0(0%)	27.7% vs. 0% at 20 years (*P*-value not documented)	Not documented	67.8% vs. 57.8% at 20 years ($P = 0.47$)

[a]Rectal cancers excluded

removed. These findings may help when surgeons select SC for patients with LS-associated first CRC. Moreover, these results may be useful for genetically proven LS patients with first CRC and their consulting surgeons to preoperatively decide the type and extent of colorectal resection.

10.3.4 Overall Survival Following SC vs. EC for First Colon Cancer and Decision Analytic Models

Two studies [5, 15] showed no significant difference in disease-free or CRC-specific survival between those who underwent SC and EC. In addition, four studies [5, 6, 15, 16] showed no significant difference in overall survival (Table 10.2). These results may be explained by the following reasons. One is that the major cause of death following surgery for first CRC is not CRC. A total of 40–61% of cancer deaths were related to extra-colonic cancers [17]. Another explanation may be the early detection of metachronous CRCs via periodic colonoscopic surveillance. Kim et al. [5] reported that 93% of patients who developed metachronous CRC presented with early-stage CRC without lymph node or systemic metastasis.

The advantage of EC may be influenced by the age at first CRC. According to the decision analysis model proposed by a Dutch study group, the overall life expectancy gain of EC (subtotal colectomy) compared with SC (hemicolectomy) at ages 27, 47, and 67 years was 2.3, 1, and 0.3 years, respectively [18]. Similarly, Syngal et al. [19] also described a decision analysis model that subtotal colectomy done at 25 years of age in patients with HNPCC led to the greatest life expectancy. Subtotal colectomy done at the time of cancer diagnosis or identification of an adenomatous polyp at an older age did not show any survival benefit compared with periodic surveillance.

Despite the low level of evidence, we should note that EC performed for first colon cancer does not lead to survival benefit compared with SC. However, EC done at young age may have significant survival benefits.

10.3.5 Risk of Metachronous Colon Cancer Following Proctectomy for First Rectal Cancer

Because of the low incidence of first rectal cancer in LS patients, we investigated the risk of metachronous CRC following rectal cancer surgery separately. Approximately 10–15% [5, 20, 21] of LS or HNPCC patients develop rectal cancer as the first CRC, and the surgical decision-making for LS patients is more complicated.

Win et al. [7] reported the results of a multinational collaborative study to evaluate the risk of metachronous CRC in 79 patients with LS (mean age, 42.8 years; range, 17–70 years) who underwent proctectomy (abdominal perineal resection in

29, anterior resection in 50) for first rectal cancer. The cumulative risk of metachronous colon cancer with a median follow-up of 9 years was 19% at 10 years, 47% at 20 years, and 69% at 30 years after proctectomy. They did not identify newly developing cancer in the remaining rectum. As described in the "Baseline characteristics of LS-associated CRC updated," 16 (76%) of the 21 metachronous CRCs were located in the right colon, which may be due to the commonly observed shift to right colon cancers in LS. Cox proportional hazard regression analysis was performed to investigate the factors influencing the risk of metachronous colon cancer and it showed that the risk of metachronous colon cancer was not associated with sex, age at rectal cancer diagnosis, country of recruitment, cigarette smoking status, maximum tumor diameter, and histologic grade of rectal cancer. However, it was associated with a higher American Joint Committee in Cancer (AJCC) stage (HR: 6.14; 95% CI: 1.21–13.14, $P = 0.03$) and the presence of synchronous tumor (HR: 11.54; 95% CI: 1.06–125, $P = 0.04$).

A pan-proctocolectomy would be theoretically a choice to eliminate the risk of metachronous CRC, particularly in patients in whom the primary tumor developed in the rectum. Thus, some surgeons might recommend IPAA as a surgical intervention due to the high risk of metachronous colon cancer following first rectal cancer surgery. However, further investigations with larger series of patients with rectal cancer are needed to determine the optimal surgical treatment for first rectal cancer in LS patients. Currently, the first rectal cancer developing in LS patients should be treated based on standard oncologic principles for sporadic rectal cancer.

10.4 Assessment for Quality of Life

To date, data on postoperative quality of life along with bowel function from different surgical procedures are incomplete. Although not limited to patients with LS, You et al. [22] compared 201 patients who underwent EC (total colectomy or subtotal colectomy) and 321 patients who underwent SC and concluded that functional outcomes regarding median daily stool frequency, urgency and looseness of stool, and quality of life including sexual relations, recreation, travel, housework, and social activity were better preserved after SC than EC. Haanstra et al. [23] surveyed patients with LS who underwent surgical treatment of CRC and compared quality of life outcomes in 51 patients who underwent SC and 53 patients who underwent EC (total colectomy) with three validated instruments. After EC, there was a detrimental effect on stool frequency, social impact, and problems with defecation. However, none of the three instruments demonstrated a negative impact on the overall quality of life between the two surgical procedures.

The extent of colectomy should therefore be balanced against functional outcomes and quality of life. Prior to surgery for first CRC, patients with LS should be informed of the functional differences and outcomes but the similar overall quality of life between the two surgical procedures.

10.5 Colonoscopic Surveillance and Chemoprevention Following Resection of First CRC

Several studies on the efficacy and interval of colonoscopic surveillance before CRC diagnosis in carriers of the LS germline pathogenic variant have been conducted. A systematic review by Lindor et al. [24] concluded that colonoscopic surveillance should be done every 1–2 years starting at age 20–25 years or at 10 years younger than the youngest age diagnosed with colon cancer in patients with a family history. Meanwhile, studies on the efficacy of postoperative colonoscopic surveillance are limited. Kalady et al. [25] reported that in a colonoscopic surveillance of 253 patients meeting the Amsterdam criteria who underwent SC, 221 (88%) of whom had postoperative surveillance at a median interval of 25 months, 55 (25%) developed metachronous CRC. Parry et al. [14] reported a 16% cumulative risk of CRC following SC at 10 years postoperatively, despite an average of 1 colonoscopy every 20 months. In addition, they reported that 47% of metachronous colon cancer following SC were diagnosed as stage I, in contrast to the study by Kalady et al. [25] that reported a higher proportion of advanced-stage disease. Although evidence is limited, annual colonoscopy has been recommended after SC by some experts [26]. Because there is clearly a risk of metachronous rectal cancer, annual colonoscopic surveillance may be recommended in patients with EC (total colectomy).

Chemoprevention in combination with stringent colonoscopic surveillance could potentially reduce the risk of metachronous CRC in patients undergoing (procto) colectomy regardless of the extent of bowel resection, but evidence is also lacking. The CAPP2 randomized controlled trial [27] demonstrated that chemoprevention with high-dose aspirin (600 mg daily) reduced the risk of developing CRC in LS patients. After a mean follow-up of 55.7 months, aspirin had a protective effect against CRC development, and the effect was even higher in those taking aspirin for 2 years or longer. This finding indicates that chemoprevention using high-dose aspirin may eliminate the need for a prophylactic extended colectomy to prevent metachronous colon cancer. However, the effect of aspirin is delayed and it is not until after a latent period of approximately a decade that the risk is significantly lowered when compared to a placebo. Despite the significant beneficial effect of aspirin, the risk of metachronous CRC following SC compared to EC seems to be already increased by several fold. Therefore, the use of high-dose aspirin is not considered as an alternative approach to EC in terms of the prevention of metachronous CRC.

10.6 Conclusions

Studies have shown that overall survival is not significantly different between EC and SC in CRC patients with LS, although EC may be a better surgical procedure than SC in terms of low risk of metachronous CRC. EC may be recommended for younger individuals with LS with CRC because it decreases the risk of metachronous CRC, leading to a survival benefit. However, several clinical factors, including the causative gene, the location of first CRC, the age of onset, the presence of synchronous tumor, and the AJCC stage, influence the development of metachronous CRC. Data on the location of first CRC and characteristics of metachronous CRC development are still limited. Particularly, whether the risk of metachronous CRC differs between patients undergoing a right-sided SC and those undergoing a left-sided SC for first colon cancer remains unclear. In addition, data on the characteristics of patients with *MHS6*, *PMS2*, or *EPCAM* variants are lacking. Thus, the optimal surgical approaches for first synchronous CRCs and metachronous CRC following SC for the first CRC are yet to be determined. The current investigation will be helpful to determine the best surgical treatment for LS patients with CRC at an individual level.

In conclusion, surgeons and patients with LS should be aware of the risk of metachronous CRC following SC despite 1–2 yearly postoperative surveillance in clinical practice. Careful preoperative counselling concerning the choice of colorectal resection for each patient is mandatory.

References

1. Edwards BK, Ward E, Kohler BA, Eheman C, Zauber AG, Anderson RN, Jemal A, Schymura MJ, Lansdorp-Vogelaar I, Seeff LC, van Ballegooijen M, Goede SL, Ries LA. Annual report to the nation on the status of cancer, 1975–2006, featuring colorectal cancer trends and impact of interventions (risk factors, screening, and treatment) to reduce future rates. Cancer. 2010;116:544–73.
2. Lynch HT, Lynch PM, Lanspa SJ, Snyder CL, Lynch JF, Boland CR. Review of the Lynch syndrome: history, molecular genetics, screening, differential diagnosis, and medicolegal ramifications. Clin Genet. 2009;76:1–18.
3. Møller P, Seppälä T, Bernstein I, Holinski-Feder E, Sala P, Evans DG, Lindblom A, Macrae F, Blanco I, Sijmons R, Jeffries J, Vasen H, Burn J, Nakken S, Hovig E, Rødland EA, Tharmaratnam K, de Vos Tot Nederveen Cappel WH, Hill J, Wijnen J, Green K, Lalloo F, Sunde L, Mints M, Bertario L, Pineda M, Navarro M, Morak M, Renkonen-Sinisalo L, Frayling IM, Plazzer JP, Pylvanainen K, Sampson JR, Capella G, Mecklin JP, Möslein G, Mallorca Group (http://mallorca-group.eu). Cancer incidence and survival in Lynch syndrome patients receiving colonoscopic and gynaecological surveillance: first report from the prospective Lynch syndrome database. Gut. 2017;66:464–72.
4. Vasen HF, Blanco I, Aktan-Collan K, Gopie JP, Alonso A, Aretz S, Bernstein I, Bertario L, Burn J, Capella G, Colas C, Engel C, Frayling IM, Genuardi M, Heinimann K, Hes FJ, Hodgson SV, Karagiannis JA, Lalloo F, Lindblom A, Mecklin JP, Møller P, Myrhoj T, Nagengast FM, Parc Y, Ponz de Leon M, Renkonen-Sinisalo L, Sampson JR, Stormorken A, Sijmons RH, Tejpar S, Thomas HJ, Rahner N, Wijnen JT, Järvinen HJ, Möslein G, Mallorca group. Revised guidelines for the clinical management of Lynch syndrome (HNPCC): recommendations by a group of European experts. Gut. 2013;62:812–23.
5. Kim TJ, Kim ER, Hong SN, Kim YH, Huh JW, Park YA, Cho YB, Yun SH, Kim HC, Lee WY, Kim K, Kim K, Chang DK. Survival outcome and risk of metachronous colorectal cancer after surgery in Lynch syndrome. Ann Surg Oncol. 2017;24:1085–92.
6. Hiatt MJ, Casey MJ, Lynch HT, Snyder CL, Stacey M, Walters RW. Efficacy of proximal colectomy for surgical management of right-sided first colorectal cancer in Lynch Syndrome mutation carriers. Am J Surg. 2018;216:99–105.
7. Win AK, Parry S, Parry B, Kalady MF, Macrae FA, Ahnen DJ, Young GP, Lipton L, Winship I, Boussioutas A, Young JP, Buchanan DD, Arnold J, Le Marchand L, Newcomb PA, Haile RW, Lindor NM, Gallinger S, Hopper JL, Jenkins MA. Risk of metachronous colon cancer

following surgery for rectal cancer in mismatch repair gene mutation carriers. Ann Surg Oncol. 2013;20:1829–36.

8. Vasen HF, Watson P, Mecklin JP, Lynch HT. New clinical criteria for hereditary nonpolyposis colorectal cancer (HNPCC, Lynch syndrome) proposed by the International Collaborative group on HNPCC. Gastroenterology. 1999;116:1453–6.
9. Heneghan HM, Martin ST, Winter DC. Segmental vs extended colectomy in the management of hereditary nonpolyposis colorectal cancer: a systematic review and meta-analysis. Color Dis. 2015;17:382–9.
10. Anele CC, Adegbola SO, Askari A, Rajendran A, Clark SK, Latchford A, Faiz OD. Risk of metachronous colorectal cancer following colectomy in Lynch syndrome: a systematic review and meta-analysis. Color Dis. 2017;19:528–36.
11. Malik SS, Lythgoe MP, McPhail M, Monahan KJ. Metachronous colorectal cancer following segmental or extended colectomy in Lynch syndrome: a systematic review and meta-analysis. Fam Cancer. 2018;17:557–64.
12. Lindor NM. Familial colorectal cancer type X: the other half of hereditary nonpolyposis colon cancer syndrome. Surg Oncol Clin N Am. 2009;18:637–45.
13. Natarajan N, Watson P, Silva-Lopez E, Lynch HT. Comparison of extended colectomy and limited resection in patients with Lynch syndrome. Dis Colon Rectum. 2010;53:77–82.
14. Parry S, Win AK, Parry B, Macrae FA, Gurrin LC, Church JM, Baron JA, Giles GG, Leggett BA, Winship I, Lipton L, Young GP, Young JP, Lodge CJ, Southey MC, Newcomb PA, Le Marchand L, Haile RW, Lindor NM, Gallinger S, Hopper JL, Jenkins MA. Metachronous colorectal cancer risk for mismatch repair gene mutation carriers: the advantage of more extensive colon surgery. Gut. 2011;60:950–7.
15. Renkonen-Sinisalo L, Seppälä TT, Järvinen HJ, Mecklin JP. Subtotal colectomy for colon cancer reduces the need for subsequent surgery in Lynch syndrome. Dis Colon Rectum. 2017;60:792–9.
16. Stupart DA, Goldberg PA, Baigrie RJ, Algar U, Ramesar R. Surgery for colonic cancer in HNPCC: total vs segmental colectomy. Color Dis. 2011;13:1395–9.
17. Pylvänäinen K, Lehtinen T, Kellokumpu I, Järvinen H, Mecklin JP. Causes of death of mutation carriers in Finnish Lynch syndrome families. Familial Cancer. 2012;11:467–71.
18. de Vos tot Nederveen Cappel WH, Buskens E, van Duijvendijk P, Cats A, Menko FH, Griffioen G, Slors JF, Nagengast FM, Kleibeuker JH, Vasen HF. Decision analysis in the surgical treatment of colorectal cancer due to a mismatch repair gene defect. Gut. 2003;52:1752–5.
19. Syngal S, Weeks JC, Schrag D, Garber JE, Kuntz KM. Benefits of colonoscopic surveillance and prophylactic colectomy in patients with hereditary nonpolyposis colorectal cancer mutations. Ann Intern Med. 1998;129:787–96.
20. Kalady MF. Surgical management of hereditary nonpolyposis colorectal cancer. Adv Surg. 2011;45:265–74.
21. Kalady MF, Lipman J, McGannon E, Church JM. Risk of colonic neoplasia after proctectomy for rectal cancer in hereditary nonpolyposis colorectal cancer. Ann Surg. 2012;255:1121–5.
22. You YN, Chua HK, Nelson H, Hassan I, Barnes SA, Harrington J. Segmental vs. extended colectomy: measurable differences in morbidity, function, and quality of life. Dis Colon Rectum. 2008;51:1036–43.
23. Haanstra JF, de Vos Tot Nederveen Cappel WH, Gopie JP, Vecht J, Vanhoutvin SA, Cats A, van der Zaag-Loonen HJ, Langers AM, Bergmann JH, van de Meeberg PC, Dekker E, Kleibeuker JH, Vasen HF, Nagengast FM, van Duijvendijk P. Quality of life after surgery for colon cancer in patients with Lynch syndrome: partial versus subtotal colectomy. Dis Colon Rectum. 2012;55:653–9.
24. Lindor NM, Petersen GM, Hadley DW, Kinney AY, Miesfeldt S, Lu KH, Lynch P, Burke W, Press N. Recommendations for the care of individuals with an inherited predisposition to Lynch syndrome: a systematic review. JAMA. 2006;296:1507–17.
25. Kalady MF, McGannon E, Vogel JD, Manilich E, Fazio VW, Church JM. Risk of colorectal adenoma and carcinoma after colectomy for colorectal cancer in patients meeting Amsterdam criteria. Ann Surg. 2010;252:507–11.

26. Herzig DO, Buie WD, Weiser MR, You YN, Rafferty JF, Feingold D, Steele SR. Clinical practice guidelines for the surgical treatment of patients with Lynch syndrome. Dis Colon Rectum. 2017;60:137–43.
27. Burn J, Gerdes AM, Macrae F, Mecklin JP, Moeslein G, Olschwang S, Eccles D, Evans DG, Maher ER, Bertario L, Bisgaard ML, Dunlop MG, Ho JW, Hodgson SV, Lindblom A, Lubinski J, Morrison PJ, Murday V, Ramesar R, Side L, Scott RJ, Thomas HJ, Vasen HF, Barker G, Crawford G, Elliott F, Movahedi M, Pylvanainen K, Wijnen JT, Fodde R, Lynch HT, Mathers JC, Bishop DT, CAPP2 Investigators. Long-term effect of aspirin on cancer risk in carriers of hereditary colorectal cancer: an analysis from the CAPP2 randomised controlled trial. Lancet. 2011;378:2081–7.

Immunotherapy for Lynch Syndrome Patients

11

Takeshi Nagasaka

Abstract

Patients with DNA mismatch repair deficient (dMMR) microsatellite instability (MSI) metastatic colorectal cancer, including Lynch syndrome, are a distinct population who benefit less from conventional chemotherapy and have a shorter overall survival than do patients with proficient MMR (pMMR) metastatic colorectal cancer. However, after the clinical breakthrough of monoclonal antibody-based immune checkpoint blockade therapies that enhance the function of antitumor T lymphocytes, the treatment of such dMMR-associated recurrent/metastatic cancers has drastically changed. This chapter aims to review some of the many advances in immunotherapy for Lynch syndrome patients with advanced cancers.

Keywords

Immune checkpoint inhibitors · Cytotoxic T-lymphocyte antigen-4 (CTLA-4) Programmed death-1 (PD-1) · Tumor mutation burden (TMB) · Frameshift peptides · Neoantigen

11.1 Immunotherapy

Immunotherapy has recently emerged as a viable and attractive cancer therapy. Monoclonal antibody-based immune checkpoint blockade therapies that enhance the function of antitumor T lymphocytes have been particularly promising, yielding unprecedented clinical efficacies. Buoyed by these successes, considerable optimism has been built in the area of immuno-oncology to capitalize on the efficacy of

T. Nagasaka (✉)
Department of Clinical Oncology, Kawasaki Medical School,
Kurashiki City, Okayama, Japan

N. Tomita (ed.), *Lynch Syndrome*, https://doi.org/10.1007/978-981-15-6891-6_11

these revolutionary cancer therapies, which have provided durable remission in many cancer patients. The concept that the immune system can recognize and control tumor progression traces its origin to 1893 when William Coley used live bacteria as an immunostimulant to treat cancer. However, restricted clinical efficacy owing to the ability of tumor cells to avoid recognition and elimination by the immune system, allowing them to become established in the host, has dampened the enthusiasm for cancer immunotherapy [1]. Over the past few decades, however, there has been tremendous progress in understanding how a cancer cell escapes the immune system, and basic research findings have enabled the development of novel approaches to halt cancer immune evasion in favor of eliminating cancer cells.

The clinical success of cancer immunotherapy has been largely achieved through immune checkpoint inhibitors (ICIs), antibodies to cytotoxic T-lymphocyte antigen-4 (CTLA-4), and programmed death-1 (PD-1) that have tipped the balance in favor of the immune system to eliminate cancer cells. These drugs work through the release of "brakes" that prevent T cells (a type of white blood cell and part of the immune system) from killing cancer cells. These drugs do not directly target the tumor, rather they interfere with the ability of cancer cells to evade an immune response. The clinical impact of cancer immunotherapy has been significant enough to warrant it being named as 2013s Breakthrough of the Year by *Science* magazine [2]. James P. Allison, who investigated CTLA-4 in an important clinical study in 2010 and showed striking effects of antibodies against CTLA-4 in patients with advanced melanoma [3–5], along with Tasuku Honjo, who discovered PD-1 and unraveled its role through a series of elegant experiments performed over several years in his laboratory at Kyoto University [6–9], received the 2018 Nobel Prize in Physiology or Medicine for their discovery of cancer therapy through inhibition of negative immune regulation.

11.2 Immune-Associated Features in Lynch Syndrome

Lynch syndrome is caused by pathogenic germline variants in the DNA mismatch repair (MMR) genes, *MLH1*, *MSH2*, *MSH6*, or *PMS2* (and, rarely, in the non-MMR gene *EPCAM*, in which deletions induce epigenetic silencing of *MSH2*) [10]. The deficiency of MMR complexes (dMMR) causes microsatellite instability (MSI), which means the somatic accumulation of small insertion or deletion events at microsatellites in the genome. When such frameshift mutations occur at hotspot microsatellite loci within coding regions of tumor suppressor genes (e.g., *TGFBR2*), they promote carcinogenesis [11]. Additionally, as these mutations generate shifts in the reading frames of many of these genes, the resulting mutant alleles often encode novel amino acid sequences, sometimes termed "frameshift peptides," some of which may function as potent tumor-specific antigens. Indeed, MSI tumors show a markedly greater presence of tumor-infiltrating lymphocytes [12, 13].

The hypothesis that dMMR/MSI tumors stimulate the immune system is not new [14]. In fact, dense immune infiltration and Th1-associated cytokine-rich environment observed in MMR-deficient tumors support the hypothesis [13, 15–18]. This has been further corroborated by a recent study showing that the dMMR tumor microenvironment strongly expressed several immune checkpoint ligands, including PD-1, PD-L1, CTLA-4, LAG-3, and IDO, indicating that the active tumor microenvironment is counterbalanced by immune inhibitory signals that resist tumor elimination [19]. The most likely explanation for these findings is that the immune infiltrate associated with dMMR carcinomas is directed at neoantigens. The correlation of a higher mutational load and a higher rate of response to anti-CTLA-4 in melanoma and anti-PD-1 in lung cancer further supports the notion that mutation-associated neoantigen recognition is an important component of the endogenous antitumor immune response [20, 21].

The Cancer Genome Atlas (TCGA) and international consensus groups have adopted consensus definitions of colorectal cancer subtypes [22], and TCGA has reported that a subset of colorectal cancers possesses markedly elevated tumor mutation burden (TMB) rates. These tumors are characterized as hypermutant phenotype based on the dysfunction of the MMR genes (most tumors in the TCGA report were sporadic MSIs) or *POLE*. Hypermutant tumors constitute a minority of colorectal cancers, with decreasing frequency in more advanced stage disease. For example, the prevalence of tumors with MSI in stage II, III, and IV colorectal cancers stand at 20%, 12%, and 4%, respectively [23–26]. Thus, Lynch syndrome-associated (and sporadic MSI) colorectal cancers have superior stage-for-stage prognoses compared with non-MSI (also termed as chromosomal instability or non-hypermutated) tumors.

11.3 ICI Therapies for Lynch Syndrome

As mentioned above, compared with patients with sporadic colorectal cancer, those with Lynch syndrome have superior stage-for-stage prognoses; however, in some cases, the latter unfortunately develop recurrent/metastatic colorectal cancer or other forms of advanced and incurable Lynch syndrome-associated cancer [27]. Targeted therapies in these individuals include monoclonal antibodies that target PD-1. In the first study of its kind to specifically examine such agents in metastatic, refractory dMMR cancers, 11 individuals with dMMR colorectal cancer, 21 individuals with MMR-proficient (pMMR) colorectal cancer, and 9 individuals with dMMR non-colorectal cancers were treated with a single-agent pembrolizumab [28]. In this cohort, there were markedly superior outcomes [hazard ratio for progression or death, 0.04; 95% confidence interval (CI), 0.01–0.21] in individuals with dMMR cancer compared with those with pMMR cancers. Overall response rates measured using RECIST criteria were 40% and 71% for dMMR colorectal cancers and non-colorectal cancers, respectively, with no responses among those with pMMR colorectal cancers. Similarly, overall disease control rates were 90% and 71% for dMMR colorectal cancers and non-colorectal cancers, respectively, compared with 11% for pMMR colorectal cancers. With a median follow-up time of 36 weeks, the median progression-free survival was not attained for either cohort of patients with dMMR cancers (vs. a median progression-free survival of only 2.2

months among patients with pMMR colorectal cancer). Follow-up data with pembrolizumab in 86 patients with a wide variety of previously treated metastatic/advanced dMMR cancers showed an objective response rate of 53% (95% CI, 42–64%) across tumor types, including a 21% complete response rate and a 77% overall disease control rate; median overall survival and progression-free survival were not attained at a median follow-up time of 12.5 months [29].

A complementary single-arm phase II study examined nivolumab, an anti-PD-1 monoclonal antibody, in 74 individuals with chemotherapy-refractory dMMR colorectal cancer [30]. An investigator-assessed objective response rate of 31.3% (23 of 74 patients) was observed in this study, and the median duration of response was not reached during the study period (median follow-up time, 12.0 months). Similarly, the median overall survival was not attained during the study period, and the median progression-free survival was 14.3 months, which indicates that the responses experienced by patients with dMMR colorectal cancer in this study were quite durable.

The use of anti-PD-1 antibodies in advanced dMMR cancers to date has not shown any significant difference in response rates or outcomes between individuals with and without known Lynch syndrome [28–30]. Correlative translational data have demonstrated marked expansion of T cells targeted toward frameshift neopeptides after treatment with anti-PD-1 antibody therapy in patients who experienced objective responses, strongly corroborating the hypothesis that these antigenic frameshift neopeptides are crucial for the success of immune-based therapies. These findings provide an impetus for strategies that leverage immune-based mechanisms to prevent Lynch syndrome-associated cancers [29]. Indeed, the response rates of ICI have been shown to positively correlate with the increase in genetic mutation number observed in cancer cells [31]. Emerging data indicate that among the primary and secondary resistance mechanisms to anti-PD-1 therapy, *β-2 microglobulin* mutations that lead to the downregulation of antigenic presentation mechanisms may account for a sizable fraction of resistance to immune checkpoint blockade [30].

These exhilarating successes led to the accelerated approval in 2017 by the US Food and Drug Administration of pembrolizumab to treat advanced, pretreated dMMR/MSI cancer (regardless of primary site) and nivolumab (dMMR/MSI colorectal cancer only). Most recently, a single-arm phase II study of nivolumab with ipilimumab (a monoclonal antibody targeted against CTLA-4) in 119 individuals with advanced dMMR/MSI colorectal cancer demonstrated an overall response rate of 55% (with 83% of all responses lasting ≥ 6 months) and a 12-month overall survival rate of 85% [32].

Furthermore, another interesting result of a study of nivolumab with ipilimumab, called the NICHE study, has been reported at ESMO2018 [33]. This study had an arm of patients with colorectal cancer without distant metastasis who underwent preoperative treatment with nivolumab with ipilimumab before surgical resection. Of the seven cases of dMMR colon cancer and eight cases of pMMR colon cancer, quite surprisingly, four out of seven cases of dMMR colon cancer showed no remnant tumor in the resected specimen (0%), and the remaining three tumor specimens showed only 1–2% remnant tumor. On the other hand, eight resected pMMR colon cancer specimens showed 85–100% remnant tumor. In the near future, dMMR colorectal cancer could be cured without surgical resection through neoadjuvant ICI therapies. These positive findings provide a fillip to synergize different mechanisms of immune checkpoint blockade to achieve tangible goals in cancer therapy.

In summary, post-ICI era, although treatment strategy is drastically changed and improved to tumors with higher mutation burden including Lynch syndrome, we should keep attention to the unnoticed evidence that ICIs do not work on all the tumors with higher mutation burden including Lynch syndrome.

References

1. Drake CG, Jaffee E, Pardoll DM. Mechanisms of immune evasion by tumors. Adv Immunol. 2006;90:51–81.
2. Couzin-Frankel J. Breakthrough of the year 2013. Cancer immunotherapy. Science. 2013;342(6165):1432–3.
3. Leach DR, Krummel MF, Allison JP. Enhancement of antitumor immunity by CTLA-4 blockade. Science. 1996;271(5256):1734–6.
4. Kwon ED, Hurwitz AA, Foster BA, Madias C, Feldhaus AL, Greenberg NM, et al. Manipulation of T cell costimulatory and inhibitory signals for immunotherapy of prostate cancer. Proc Natl Acad Sci U S A. 1997;94(15):8099–103.
5. Hodi FS, Mihm MC, Soiffer RJ, Haluska FG, Butler M, Seiden MV, et al. Biologic activity of cytotoxic T lymphocyte-associated antigen 4 antibody blockade in previously vaccinated metastatic melanoma and ovarian carcinoma patients. Proc Natl Acad Sci U S A. 2003;100(8):4712–7.
6. Ishida Y, Agata Y, Shibahara K, Honjo T. Induced expression of PD-1, a novel member of the immunoglobulin gene superfamily, upon programmed cell death. EMBO J. 1992;11(11):3887–95.
7. Nishimura H, Nose M, Hiai H, Minato N, Honjo T. Development of lupus-like autoimmune diseases by disruption of the PD-1 gene encoding an ITIM motif-carrying immunoreceptor. Immunity. 1999;11(2):141–51.
8. Freeman GJ, Long AJ, Iwai Y, Bourque K, Chernova T, Nishimura H, et al. Engagement of the PD-1 immunoinhibitory receptor by a novel B7 family member leads to negative regulation of lymphocyte activation. J Exp Med. 2000;192(7):1027–34.
9. Iwai Y, Terawaki S, Honjo T. PD-1 blockade inhibits hematogenous spread of poorly immunogenic tumor cells by enhanced recruitment of effector T cells. Int Immunol. 2005;17(2):133–44.
10. Yurgelun MB, Hampel H. Recent advances in Lynch syndrome: diagnosis, treatment, and cancer prevention. Am Soc Clin Oncol Educ Book. 2018;38:101–9.
11. Spira A, Disis ML, Schiller JT, Vilar E, Rebbeck TR, Bejar R, et al. Leveraging premalignant biology for immune-based cancer prevention. Proc Natl Acad Sci U S A. 2016;113(39):10750–8.
12. Kloor M, von Knebel Doeberitz M. The immune biology of microsatellite-unstable cancer. Trends Cancer. 2016;2(3):121–33.
13. Smyrk TC, Watson P, Kaul K, Lynch HT. Tumor-infiltrating lymphocytes are a marker for microsatellite instability in colorectal carcinoma. Cancer. 2001;91(12):2417–22.
14. Bodmer W, Bishop T, Karran P. Genetic steps in colorectal cancer. Nat Genet. 1994;6(3):217–9.
15. Dolcetti R, Viel A, Doglioni C, Russo A, Guidoboni M, Capozzi E, et al. High prevalence of activated intraepithelial cytotoxic T lymphocytes and increased neoplastic cell apoptosis in colorectal carcinomas with microsatellite instability. Am J Pathol. 1999;154(6):1805–13.
16. Alexander J, Watanabe T, Wu TT, Rashid A, Li S, Hamilton SR. Histopathological identification of colon cancer with microsatellite instability. Am J Pathol. 2001;158(2):527–35.

17. Young J, Simms LA, Biden KG, Wynter C, Whitehall V, Karamatic R, et al. Features of colorectal cancers with high-level microsatellite instability occurring in familial and sporadic settings: parallel pathways of tumorigenesis. Am J Pathol. 2001;159(6):2107–16.
18. Kim H, Jen J, Vogelstein B, Hamilton SR. Clinical and pathological characteristics of sporadic colorectal carcinomas with DNA replication errors in microsatellite sequences. Am J Pathol. 1994;145(1):148–56.
19. Llosa NJ, Cruise M, Tam A, Wicks EC, Hechenbleikner EM, Taube JM, et al. The vigorous immune microenvironment of microsatellite instable colon cancer is balanced by multiple counter-inhibitory checkpoints. Cancer Discov. 2015;5(1):43–51.
20. Snyder A, Makarov V, Merghoub T, Yuan J, Zaretsky JM, Desrichard A, et al. Genetic basis for clinical response to CTLA-4 blockade in melanoma. N Engl J Med. 2014;371(23):2189–99.
21. Rizvi NA, Hellmann MD, Snyder A, Kvistborg P, Makarov V, Havel JJ, et al. Cancer immunology. Mutational landscape determines sensitivity to PD-1 blockade in non-small cell lung cancer. Science. 2015;348(6230):124–8.
22. The Cancer Genome Atlas Network. Comprehensive molecular characterization of human colon and rectal cancer. Nature. 2012;487(7407):330–7.
23. Raut CP, Pawlik TM, Rodriguez-Bigas MA. Clinicopathologic features in colorectal cancer patients with microsatellite instability. Mutat Res. 2004;568(2):275–82.
24. Hampel H, Frankel WL, Martin E, Arnold M, Khanduja K, Kuebler P, et al. Screening for the Lynch syndrome (hereditary nonpolyposis colorectal cancer). N Engl J Med. 2005;352(18):1851–60.
25. Koopman M, Kortman GA, Mekenkamp L, Ligtenberg MJ, Hoogerbrugge N, Antonini NF, et al. Deficient mismatch repair system in patients with sporadic advanced colorectal cancer. Br J Cancer. 2009;100(2):266–73.
26. Vilar E, Tabernero J. Molecular dissection of microsatellite instable colorectal cancer. Cancer Discov. 2013;3(5):502–11.
27. Sankila R, Aaltonen LA, Jarvinen HJ, Mecklin JP. Better survival rates in patients with MLH1-associated hereditary colorectal cancer. Gastroenterology. 1996;110(3):682–7.
28. Le DT, Uram JN, Wang H, Bartlett BR, Kemberling H, Eyring AD, et al. PD-1 blockade in tumors with mismatch-repair deficiency. N Engl J Med. 2015;372(26):2509–20.
29. Le DT, Durham JN, Smith KN, Wang H, Bartlett BR, Aulakh LK, et al. Mismatch repair deficiency predicts response of solid tumors to PD-1 blockade. Science. 2017;357(6349):409–13.
30. Overman MJ, McDermott R, Leach JL, Lonardi S, Lenz HJ, Morse MA, et al. Nivolumab in patients with metastatic DNA mismatch repair-deficient or microsatellite instability-high colorectal cancer (CheckMate 142): an open-label, multicentre, phase 2 study. Lancet Oncol. 2017;18(9):1182–91.
31. Yarchoan M, Hopkins A, Jaffee EM. Tumor mutational burden and response rate to PD-1 inhibition. N Engl J Med. 2017;377(25):2500–1.
32. Overman MJ, Lonardi S, Wong KYM, Lenz HJ, Gelsomino F, Aglietta M, et al. Durable clinical benefit with nivolumab plus ipilimumab in DNA mismatch repair-deficient/microsatellite instability-high metastatic colorectal cancer. J Clin Oncol. 2018;36(8):773–9.
33. Chalabi M, Fanchi LF, Van den Berg JG, Beets GL, Lopez-Yurda M, Aalbers AG, Grootscholten C, Snaebjornsson P, Maas M, Mertz M, Nuijten E, Kuiper M, Kok M, Van Leerdam ME, Schumacher TN, Voest EE, Haanen JB. Neoadjuvant ipilimumab plus nivolumab in early stage colon cancer. ESMO2018. 2018.

Chemoprevention for Lynch Syndrome-Associated Malignancies

12

Michihiro Mutoh, Takumi Narita, and Hideki Ishikawa

Abstract

Recently, patients who have been diagnosed with colorectal cancer (CRC) at a younger age are increasing and display more hereditary CRC than previously thought. The development of next-generation sequencing gene panel testing will diagnose more patients; thus, the number of Lynch syndrome (LS) patients may increase in the future. As a result, we must perform CRC screening and target preventive measures to younger individuals. In addition to diet and lifestyle modifications that encompass cancer prevention, cancer chemopreventive agents have been adopted for those who are in high-risk cancer groups, such as LS. The routine use of chemopreventive agents for patients with LS remains under debate. However, aspirin chemoprevention trials for LS-associated CRC

M. Mutoh (✉)
Department of Molecular-Targeting Prevention, Kyoto Prefectural University of Medicine, Kyoto, Japan

Epidemiology and Prevention Division, Research Center for Cancer Prevention and Screening, National Cancer Center, Tokyo, Japan

Carcinogenesis and Cancer Prevention Division, National Cancer Center Research Institute, Tokyo, Japan
e-mail: mimutoh@koto.kpu-m.ac.jp

T. Narita
Department of Molecular-Targeting Prevention, Kyoto Prefectural University of Medicine, Kyoto, Japan

Epidemiology and Prevention Division, Research Center for Cancer Prevention and Screening, National Cancer Center, Tokyo, Japan

H. Ishikawa
Department of Molecular-Targeting Prevention, Kyoto Prefectural University of Medicine, Kyoto, Japan

N. Tomita (ed.), *Lynch Syndrome*, https://doi.org/10.1007/978-981-15-6891-6_12

yielded promising results for future clinical use. In this chapter, we introduce cancer chemoprevention and focus on the current status and future prospects of chemoprevention for LS-associated malignancies.

Keywords

Chemoprevention · Lynch syndrome · Colorectal cancer · Aspirin · Trials

12.1 Introduction

In this chapter, important aspects of the current status and future prospects for cancer chemoprevention against Lynch syndrome (LS)-associated malignancies are summarized.

12.1.1 Chemoprevention

Chemoprevention was first introduced by Dr. Sporn in 1976 [1]. Chemoprevention is now defined as the ability to suppress, delay, or reverse carcinogenesis and the resultant prevention of cancer development by the use of specific agents, including natural and chemical compounds [2]. This term is applied to agents that could also play a role in several carcinogenesis steps. Cancer chemopreventive agents are expected to possess a function, such as blocking the action of carcinogenic agents that change DNA, activating the DNA repair system, decreasing cell cycle speed or inhibiting the spread of cancer through metastasis [3].

12.1.2 Subjects Adopted for Cancer Chemoprevention

As the user of cancer chemopreventive agents is not a cancer patient, the ideal cancer chemopreventive agent must meet several criteria, such as a convenient dosing schedule, easy administration, low cost, and low side effects. Cancer chemopreventive agents are adopted for those who are in cancer high-risk groups. Recently, chemoprevention has been used for those who already have cancer but are not showing clinical symptoms or who have premalignant/precursor lesions. Generally, cancer chemopreventive agents are not adopted for the general population. The highest return from chemopreventive strategies may be in patients with a hereditary predisposition for developing colorectal cancer (CRC). Among familial gastrointestinal cancer syndromes [4], familial adenomatous polyposis (FAP), and Lynch syndrome (LS) may fall under this consideration. FAP is a rare autosomal dominant inherited disorder mainly attributed to *APC* gene mutation and typically characterized by the occurrence of more than 100 polyps in the colorectum and other parts of the intestine. Half of FAP patients develop CRC by the age of 40 [5]. Patients with LS, also called a hereditary non-polyposis colon cancer (HNPCC), develop malignant lesions due to a breakdown of the DNA mismatch repair (MMR) gene. Notably, there are other polyposis syndromes, such as juvenile polyposis, in which the responsible gene is *SMAD4*, Peutz Jeghers syndrome, in which the responsible gene is *STK11*, and Cowden syndrome, in which the responsible gene is *PTEN*.

12.1.3 Sources of Finding Chemopreventive Agents

The development of cancer chemopreventive agents in LS is discussed in a separate section. In this report, we describe the sources of developing common cancer chemopreventive agents. The identification of chemopreventive agents comes from different sources: (1) data from observation studies demonstrating that specific eating habits have lower incidences of specific cancers, (2) data from epidemiological studies or clinical studies that improved cancer outcomes in a study population as a secondary effect of a drug, and (3) data from laboratory studies showing the use of an agent not only inhibits cell proliferation but also elicits surrogate markers of a malignant to normal reversion at some level [6].

12.1.4 Recent Results of Cancer Chemoprevention Studies

A decrease in cell count or cell proliferation in cancerous cells by candidates of cancer chemopreventive agents in the laboratory can be easily observed, but it is not easy to demonstrate the chemopreventive properties of potential agents when trials are performed on the populations. Thus, to date, the results of cancer chemoprevention are more scarcer than expected. Although a large number of candidates of chemopreventive agents have already been tested, in the USA, there are only approximately 15 molecules approved by the US Food and Drug Administration (FDA) for use as cancer chemopreventive agents [3]. For instance, tamoxifen and raloxifene, a selective antagonist of the estrogen receptor, have been approved for breast cancer, aspirin and celecoxib have been approved for CRC, and the human papillomavirus (HPV) vaccine has been approved for cervical cancer. Tamoxifen is the first chemopreventive agent approved by the FDA and it works because a high proportion of breast cancers express estrogen receptors that cause cancer cell proliferation. We have found recent ongoing trials that successfully achieved translational research in public trial registries (https://www.ClinicalTrials.gov/, www.ISRCTN.com, www.umin.ac.jp/ctr/index/htm, or www.trialregister.nl).

12.1.5 Chemoprevention for Colorectal Cancer

In the case of CRC prevention, treatment should ultimately be aimed at delaying colectomy, reducing frequent performance of endoscopies and polypectomies and preventing cancer development.

Based on reports of chemopreventive activity in the literature and/or efficacy data from in vivo and in vitro models, the most promising drugs that prevent CRC are aspirin and other nonsteroidal anti-inflammatory drugs (NSAIDs) [7, 8]. The FDA approved aspirin and celecoxib for adults aged 50–59 with a higher risk of CRC and individuals greater than 18 years old from FAP families, respectively. The effectiveness of these drugs may be attributed to the inhibition of cyclooxygenase (COX) enzyme activity. Another agent that possesses anti-inflammatory function is omega-3 polyunsaturated fatty acid, which has been proven to inhibit carcinogenesis in FAP patients [9]. However, there is a possibility of a drawback in serum-free fatty acids that may induce cells less sensitive to insulin and thus promote hyperglycemia [10]. In the case of metformin, a biguanide compound used for the treatment of diabetes mellitus, and statins, which are used for lowering cholesterol, the results are both still controversial. Recently, chemopreventive effects of metformin on sporadic adenoma recurrence were shown by a double-blind, placebo-controlled, randomized trial [11]. Further studies are needed to confirm the robust evidence collected from this trial.

12.2 Chemoprevention Trial for Lynch Syndrome

The routine use of chemopreventive agents for patients with LS remains debated. However, there are several chemoprevention trials for LS using aspirin, calcium supplementation ($CaCO_3$), sulindac, celecoxib, and other agents [12]. Among these agents, aspirin seems to be of real interest. Calcium and sulindac failed to obtain positive results. We will introduce several chemoprevention trials for LS including ongoing trials.

12.2.1 Aspirin Trial

12.2.1.1 CAPP2

The regular use of aspirin or other NSAIDs has been reported to reduce the risk of colorectal adenomas and cancer. In addition, resistant starch has also been reported to show antineoplastic effects on rodent carcinogenesis models [13, 14]. However, the utility of aspirin, resistant starch or both have been unknown in terms of whether they will prevent colorectal carcinogenesis in LS before the Colorectal Adenoma/Carcinoma Prevention Program (CAPP) 2 trial.

The CAPP2 trial is the largest chemoprevention trial for LS-associated CRC. Another feature of this trial is that it is the first double-blind randomized trial of aspirin chemoprevention with LS-associated CRC as a primary endpoint. This trial is designed as a 2 × 2 factorial randomized trial. Lynch syndrome gene carriers (n = 861) were divided into intervention groups of an aspirin enteric-coated tablet (600 mg/day for a minimum of 2 years), resistant starch (30 g/day for a minimum of 2 years), and a matched placebo (427 participants) for 1–4 years. This trial has also planned a 10-year follow-up [15]. The primary endpoint of this trial was detection of more than one colorectal adenoma or CRC. Secondary endpoints were the detection of an adenoma only, CRC only and advanced adenoma or CRC.

After a mean observation period of 29 months, aspirin was not shown to affect the development of colorectal neoplasia. However, after a longer observation period of 55.7 months, LS patients treated with 600 mg/day aspirin for at least 2 years showed a hazard ratio of 0.63 (CI 0.35–1.13 $P = 0.02$) for LS-associated CRC compared to the placebo. Adverse events in the aspirin and placebo group were almost the same. Other findings from CAPP2 are that obesity is associated with a substantially increased CRC risk. The risk in the obese LS participants was 2.41 × (95% CI, 1.22–4.85) greater than for underweight and normal-weight participants [16]. Interestingly, this risk is abrogated by taking aspirin. Findings from CAPP2 suggest that a follow-up for several years after a randomized trial might be necessary to evaluate the effects of aspirin and other CRC chemopreventive agents.

12.2.1.2 CAPP3

To recommend the routine use of aspirin in LS patients, the optimal aspirin dose, duration of use, and aspirin-associated side effects must be further evaluated. Notably, 600 mg doses of aspirin are not available in the USA. Therefore, the CAPP3 trial aims to randomize 1000 LS mutation carriers to three doses of aspirin (100, 300 and 600 mg/day) and will examine the CRC incidence and adverse event rate during the 5–10-year follow-up period [17]. This CAPP3 trial is currently ongoing.

12.2.1.3 AAS-Lynch

Another clinical trial (AAS-Lynch) will evaluate the effect of low-dose aspirin (100 mg/day or 300 mg/day) for 4 years on colorectal adenoma formation in 18–75-year-old LS patients. The primary endpoint of this trial is the number of patients with at least one adenoma seen on chromo-endoscopy 48 months after complete withdrawal of polyps and initiation of treatment (aspirin or placebo). This AAS-Lynch trial (NCT02813824) is also currently ongoing.

12.2.2 Naproxen Trial

In the mouse model of LS, it has been shown that naproxen is a more effective chemopreventive agent than aspirin. Similar to aspirin, naproxen is an NSAID with minimal cardiac side effects. This randomized phase Ib/II clinical trial (NCT02052908) is investigating the effects of naproxen in preventing LS-associated CRC. This study investigates the safety of naproxen by examining side effects, such as ulcer, heart attack, and kidney disorders, and the change of the molecule in the normal colonic mucosa by naproxen treatment. Patients receive high-dose naproxen (440 mg/day), low-dose naproxen (220 mg/day), or placebo for 6 months [18]. The dose of naproxen is equivalent to the recommended amount on the market (1 tablet or 2 tablets of 220 mg tablets). Participants undergo colonoscopy before treatment and 6 months after treatment. Prostaglandin E_2 levels will be measured from participants' blood, urine, and tissue samples. Moreover, the effects of long-term naproxen treatment on tissues, messenger RNA and microRNA signatures will be assessed. Similar to the aspirin, this trial attempting to discover biomarkers to identify the most effective subjects for naproxen.

12.2.3 Progestin Trial

Endometrial cancer, breast cancer, and ovarian cancer are presumed to be an estrogen-driven malignancy. Observational and case control studies showed that the use of progestin-containing oral contraceptive pills (OCPs) has been associated with a reduction of endometrial cancer risk in the general population [19, 20].

A short-term phase II randomized chemoprevention study was performed to investigate the effects of progestin-containing OCPs or depo-medroxyprogesterone acetate (depoMPA) on endometrial proliferation in women with LS [21]. Asymptomatic women (25–50 years old) with a diagnosis of LS underwent baseline transvaginal ultrasound and endometrial biopsy and were then randomized to the two groups that receive progestin-containing OCPs or depoMPA for 3 months followed by repeat transvaginal ultrasound and endometrial biopsy. A total of 51 women were enrolled, and 46 completed the treatment. The primary endpoint was change in endometrial proliferation measured by Ki67 expression on endometrial biopsies performed pre- and posttreatment. Secondary endpoints were changes in endometrial histology, endometrial thickness, and expression of estrogen-modulated genes. These results demonstrated that women with LS showed an endometrial response to short-term exogenous progestin exposure.

12.3 Chemoprevention for LS in the Future

As mentioned in the previous section, clinical trials to prevent cancer with LS have not been sufficiently performed, and aspirin is the only promising drug at the present time. Pharmacoepidemiological data on LS are not present at the moment. Therefore, to increase the number of candidates of cancer chemopreventive agents, it is necessary to begin drug screening in cells and conduct animal experiments.

Isolating products or plant extracts that are not toxic for continuous human consumption is a challenge, and the difficulty is very significant in translational medicine. Thus, it is important to include ideas of drug repositioning because information on side effects is already examined for medicines before their development. The ideal compound for chemoprevention is as follows: one that (1) has little or no toxicity, (2) presents high efficacy, (3) can be taken orally, (4) has a known mechanism of action, (5) is a low-cost drug, and (6) displays easy human acceptance for the years in which it is taken. It will be helpful when screening drugs with to keep these points in mind.

Even in aspirin, a safe medicine with long accepted use, the proper doses and when it should start being used as a chemopreventive agent lead to discussions. In LS patients, a benefit will be seen when with aspirin use, but higher doses and continuous use might be related to gastric and intracranial hemorrhages. It is desirable to prepare guidelines to select LS patients who show aspirin chemopreventive effects and are less likely to have side effects.

12.3.1 Establishment of Screening Method for LS-Associated Colorectal Cancer

LS is a disease in which cancer occurs due to gene instability as a result of a pathogenic mutation in one of four MMR genes: *MLH1*, *MSH2*, *MSH6*, or *PMS2*. Inactivation of the *MSH* or *MLH* genes are driven by methylation rather than mutation. *MLH1* and *MSH2* mutations are responsible for greater than 90% of all cases of LS [22]. Those errors tend to occur in microsatellite areas. Thus, the molecular hallmark of LS cancers is this high microsatellite instability (MSI), which is present in approximately 93% of tumors [23].

MMR-deficient cells are adequate models to investigate LS-associated CRC in vitro. Some of the MMR-deficient human CRC cell lines are as follows: HCT116 (*MLH1*, base substitution resulting in a termination signal at exon 9 codon 252), SW48 (*MLH1*, promoter methylation), RKO (*MLH1*, promoter methylation), HCT15/DLD1 (*MSH6*, 1 bp deletion at codon 222 resulting in a nonsense mutation and frameshift mutation at codon 1103 that causes a new stop colon 9 bp downstream) [12].

Our group has developed an in vitro screening system to develop an effective cancer chemopreventive agent for FAP patients. FAP is also involved in familial gastrointestinal cancer syndromes. In this in vitro screening method, we focused on three signaling pathways that may be involved in the early stages of colon carcinogenesis (Wnt, NF-κB, NRF2) and selected agents that inhibit TCF/LEF and NF-κB and activate NRF2 transcriptional activity in several human CRC cells. Aberration of Wnt signaling is assumed to be the first step in the colorectal carcinogenic process, regardless of chromosomal instability (CIN) or MSI. Of note, almost 90% of colorectal cancer is associated with activated Wnt signaling through mutations of *APC* and/or *CTNNB1* (beta-catenin). Conversely, mutation signature analysis in LS-associated CRC revealed that *KRAS* and *APC* mutations commonly occur after the onset of MMR deficiency [24]. Thus, we believe that an in vitro screening method for FAP could be used for LS-associated CRC. Indeed, our idea is supported by the observation that aspirin, which is useful to prevent colorectal tumor in FAP patients [8], at doses ≥325 mg/day reduced the incidence of LS-associated CRC by >50% [25]. These results are encouraging from the point of view that inhibition of inflammation status may be an effective chemopreventive strategy in typical *APC*-mediated tumors/adenomas and lesions with an MSI phenotype.

12.3.2 Establishment of Animal Models for LS-Associated Colorectal Cancer

Using precursor lesions, such as colorectal adenoma, for developing chemopreventive agents is an attractive method. However, it is important to develop animal models in which these lesions are developed and could be easily monitored for progression to cancer or response to intervention.

Familial gastrointestinal cancer syndromes in genetically engineered mice models are well summarized elsewhere [26]. Mouse models for MMR genes, such as *Mlh1, Msh2, Msh6, and Pms2*, have been under investigation for many years. Heterozygous knockout of the *Mlh* or *Msh* genes failed to show a cancer phenotype [26]. Homozygous knockout of the *Mlh* or *Msh* genes develop small intestine tumors, but lymphomas are also developed. The intestinal tumors showed MSI and as expected, routinely exhibited mutations in *Apc*. Loss of APC function seems to play a critical role for cancer development in an MMR-deficient genetic background. Concomitant mutation in MMR genes and the *Apc* allele ($Apc^{Min/+}$ or $Apc^{1638N/+}$ mice) results in accelerated tumorigenesis and limits tumor development in the intestinal tract [27]. In the case of LS-associated CRC with an *APC* mutation, these mouse models provide an excellent tool for studying novel chemopreventive agents. Another mouse model with a mutation in MMR genes and mutations in *TgfβRII* or *Bax* is desired to further understand LS-associated CRC.

12.4 Future Aspects

Clearly, benefits from diet and lifestyle modification targeting cancer prevention should be considered before advancing cancer chemoprevention to high-risk individuals. Physical activity, weight control, low-fat diet, consumption of abundant fruits and vegetables and smoking cessation have all been robustly demonstrated to prevent cancer. This preventive method is useful not only for the prevention of cancer but also for the prevention of other chronic diseases. There are no drugs without side effects that depend on the dose and time of use. Thus, a risk/benefit consideration should be made in order to decide whether a chemopreventive agent should be used [28].

The development of next-generation sequencing gene panel testing will improve the ability to diagnose more patients. Recently, in the USA, patients who are diagnosed with CRC at a younger age display more hereditary CRC than has previously been thought [29]. In addition, CRC incidence trends in Surveillance, Epidemiology, and End Result areas from 1974 to 2013 ($n = 490\ 305$) revealed that the incidence of CRC in young individuals continues to rise [30]. These data imply that the number of LS patients may increase in the future, and we must perform CRC screening and target preventative measures to individuals younger than 50 years of age.

The next-generation panel testing will define the exact mutations, and a precise genetic diagnosis for LS enables a better understanding of the nuances between different gene mutations, the relevance of some variants, and the spectrum of the syndrome. These results may help to identify nongenetic modifiers that may influence the clinical phenotype of LS in basic research and help to design cancer chemoprevention trials that may be successfully conducted without wasting resources and time.

References

1. Sung JJ, Lau JY, Goh KL, Leung WK, Asia Pacific Working Group on Colorectal Cancer. Increasing incidence of colorectal cancer in Asia: implications for screening. Lancet Oncol. 2005;6:871–6.
2. Tomasetti C, Vogelstein B. Cancer etiology. Variation in cancer risk among tissues can be explained by the number of stem cell divisions. Science. 2015;347:78–81.
3. de Melo FHM, Oliveira JS, Sartorelli VOB, Montor WR. Cancer chemoprevention: classic and epigenetic mechanisms inhibiting tumorigenesis. What have we learned so far? Front Oncol. 2018;8:644.
4. Lynch HT, Lynch JF, Shaw TG. Hereditary gastrointestinal cancer syndromes. Gastrointest Cancer Res. 2011;4:S9–S17.
5. Iwama T, Tamura K, Morita T, Hirai T, Hasegawa H, Koizumi K, Shirouzu K, Sugihara K, Yamamura T, Muto T, Utsunomiya J, Japanese Society for Cancer of the Colon and Rectum. A clinical overview of familial adenomatous polyposis derived from the database of the Polyposis Registry of Japan. Int J Clin Oncol. 2004;9:308–16.
6. Patterson SL, Colbert Maresso K, Hawk E. Cancer chemoprevention: successes and failures. Clin Chem. 2013;59:94–101.
7. Ishikawa H, Mutoh M, Suzuki S, Tokudome S, Saida Y, Abe T, Okamura S, Tajika M, Joh T, Tanaka S, Kudo S, Matsuda T, Iimuro M, Yukawa T, Takayama T, Sato Y, Lee K, Kitamura S, Mizuno M, Sano Y, Gondo N, Sugimoto K, Kusunoki M, Goto C, Matsuura N, Sakai T, Wakabayashi K. The preventive effects of low-dose enteric-coated aspirin tablets on the development of colorectal tumours in Asian patients: a randomized trial. Gut. 2014;63:1755–9.
8. Ishikawa H, Wakabayashi K, Suzuki S, Mutoh M, Hirata K, Nakamura T, Takeyama I, Kawano A, Gondo N, Abe T, Tokudome S, Goto C, Matsuura N, Sakai T. Preventive effects of low-dose aspirin on colorectal adenoma growth in patients with familial adenomatous polyposis: double-blind, randomized clinical trial. Cancer Med. 2013;2:50–6.
9. West NJ, Clark SK, Phillips RK, Hutchinson JM, Leicester RJ, Belluzzi A, Hull MA. Eicosapentaenoic acid reduces rectal polyp number and size in familial adenomatous polyposis. Gut. 2010;59:918–25.
10. Serhan CN, Hong S, Gronert K, Colgan SP, Devchand PR, Mirick G, Moussignac RL. Resolvins: a family of bioactive products of omega-3 fatty acid transformation circuits initiated by aspirin treatment that counter proinflammation signals. J Exp Med. 2002;196:1025–37.
11. Higurashi T, Hosono K, Takahashi H, Komiya Y, Umezawa S, Sakai E, Uchiyama T, Taniguchi L, Hata Y, Uchiyama S, Hattori A, Nagase H, Kessoku T, Arimoto J, Matsuhashi N, Inayama Y, Yamanaka S, Taguri M, Nakajima A. Metformin for chemoprevention of metachronous colorectal adenoma or polyps in post-polypectomy patients without diabetes: a multicentre double-blind, placebo-controlled, randomised phase 3 trial. Lancet Oncol. 2016;17:475–83.
12. Heijink DM, de Vries EG, Koornstra JJ, Hospers GA, Hofstra RM, van Vugt MA, de Jong S, Kleibeuker JH. Perspectives for tailored chemoprevention and treatment of colorectal cancer in Lynch syndrome. Crit Rev Oncol Hematol. 2011;80:264–77.
13. Pierre F, Perrin P, Champ M, Bornet F, Meflah K, Menanteau J. Short-chain fructo-oligosaccharides reduce the occurrence of colon tumors and develop gut-associated lymphoid tissue in Min mice. Cancer Res. 1997;57:225–8.
14. Nelson B, Cray N, Ai Y, Fang Y, Liu P, Whitley EM, Birt D. Effect of dietary-resistant starch on inhibition of colonic preneoplasia and Wnt signaling in azoxymethane-induced rodent models. Nutr Cancer. 2016;68:1052–63.

15. Burn J, Gerdes AM, Macrae F, Mecklin JP, Moeslein G, Olschwang S, Eccles D, Evans DG, Maher ER, Bertario L, Bisgaard ML, Dunlop MG, Ho JW, Hodgson SV, Lindblom A, Lubinski J, Morrison PJ, Murday V, Ramesar R, Side L, Scott RJ, Thomas HJ, Vasen HF, Barker G, Crawford G, Elliott F, Movahedi M, Pylvanainen K, Wijnen JT, Fodde R, Lynch HT, Mathers JC, Bishop DT, CAPP2 Investigators. Long-term effect of aspirin on cancer risk in carriers of hereditary colorectal cancer: an analysis from the CAPP2 randomised controlled trial. Lancet. 2011;378:2081–7.
16. Movahedi M, Bishop DT, Macrae F, Mecklin JP, Moeslein G, Olschwang S, Eccles D, Evans DG, Maher ER, Bertario L, Bisgaard ML, Dunlop MG, Ho JW, Hodgson SV, Lindblom A, Lubinski J, Morrison PJ, Murday V, Ramesar RS, Side L, Scott RJ, Thomas HJ, Vasen HF, Burn J, Mathers JC. Obesity, aspirin, and risk of colorectal cancer in carriers of hereditary colorectal cancer: a prospective investigation in the CAPP2 Study. J Clin Oncol. 2015;33:3591–7.
17. Burn J, Sheth H. The role of aspirin in preventing colorectal cancer. Br Med Bull. 2016;119:17–24.
18. Begum R, Martin SA. Targeting mismatch repair defects: a novel strategy for personalized cancer treatment. DNA Repair. 2016;38:135–9.
19. Weiss NS, Sayvetz TA. Incidence of endometrial cancer in relation to the use of oral contraceptives. N Engl J Med. 1980;302:551–4.
20. Hannaford PC, Selvaraj S, Elliott AM, Angus V, Iversen L, Lee AJ. Cancer risk among users of oral contraceptives: cohort data from the Royal College of General Practitioner's oral contraception study. BMJ. 2007;335:651.
21. Lu KH, Loose DS, Yates MS, Nogueras-Gonzalez GM, Munsell MF, Chen LM, Lynch H, Cornelison T, Boyd-Rogers S, Rubin M, Daniels MS, Conrad P, Milbourne A, Gershenson DM, Broaddus RR. Prospective, multi-center randomized intermediate biomarker study of oral contraceptive vs. Depo-Provera for prevention of endometrial cancer in women with Lynch syndrome. Cancer Prev Res. 2013;6:774–81.
22. de la Chapelle A. The incidence of Lynch syndrome. Familial Cancer. 2005;4:233–7.
23. Möslein G, Nelson H, Thibodeau S, Dozois RR. Rectal carcinomas in HNPCC. Langenbecks Arch Chir Suppl Kongressbd. 1998;115:1467–9.
24. Ahadova A, Gallon R, Gebert J, Ballhausen A, Endris V, Kirchner M, Stenzinger A, Burn J, von Knebel DM, Bläker H, Kloor M. Three molecular pathways model colorectal carcinogenesis in Lynch syndrome. Int J Cancer. 2018;143:139–50.
25. Langley RE, Rothwell PM. Aspirin in gastrointestinal oncology: new data on an old friend. Curr Opin Oncol. 2014;26:441–7.
26. Jahid S, Lipkin S. Mouse models of inherited cancer syndromes. Hematol Oncol Clin North Am. 2010;24:1205–28.
27. Taketo MM, Edelmann W. Mouse models of colon cancer. Gastroenterology. 2009;136:780–98.
28. Kotecha R, Takami A, Espinoza JL. Dietary phytochemicals and cancer chemoprevention: a review of the clinical evidence. Oncotarget. 2016;7:52517–29.
29. Mork ME, You YN, Ying J, Bannon SA, Lynch PM, Rodriguez-Bigas MA, Vilar E. High prevalence of hereditary cancer syndromes in adolescents and young adults with colorectal cancer. J Clin Oncol. 2015;33:3544–9.
30. Siegel RL, Fedewa SA, Anderson WF, Miller KD, Ma J, Rosenberg PS, Jemal A. Colorectal cancer incidence patterns in the United States, 1974–2013. J Natl Cancer Inst. 2017;109:djw322.

International Collaboration for Lynch Syndrome

13

Nagahide Matsubara

Abstract

Lynch syndrome (LS) is a common hereditary colorectal cancer (CRC) syndrome, however the diagnosis of LS in daily clinical practice is still difficult due to the insignificant manifestation of the disease compared to other hereditary CRCs such as FAP, which typically develops thousands of polyps in a large intestine and simply identified by colonoscopy. International collaboration is always essential in understanding of the etiology and the clinical manifestations of the rare diseases such as hereditary cancer syndromes. International collaboration group for LS was established as an ICG-HNPCC (International collaborative group on hereditary non-polyposis colorectal cancer) and the first meeting was held at Amsterdam hosted by Hans Vasen in 1990. ICG-HNPCC merged to Leeds Castle Polyposis Group (LCPG) and the International Society for Gastrointestinal Hereditary Tumors (InSiGHT) was established in 2005. This society was always the center of the physician, surgeon, researcher, geneticist, genetic counselor, etc. involved in this field and established clinical criteria and central database with collection of causative gene alterations for clinical use. It also supported multiple international research collaborations. Other related collaboration groups such as European Hereditary Tumor Group and Collaborative Group of the Americans on Inherited Gastrointestinal Cancer (CGA-IGC) are also mentioned.

Keywords

Lynch syndrome · Hereditary cancer · Colorectal cancer · International collaboration · Hereditary non-polyposis colorectal cancer

---

N. Matsubara (✉)
Amagasaki Chuou Hospital, Aamagasaki, Hyogo, Japan
e-mail: n-matsubara@chuoukai.or.jp

N. Tomita (ed.), *Lynch Syndrome*, https://doi.org/10.1007/978-981-15-6891-6_13

13.1 Introduction

Individual energetic work is important in understanding unknown disease or syndrome, however collaboration especially international collaboration is always essential in understanding of the etiology and the clinical manifestations of the rare diseases such as hereditary cancer syndromes. Although Lynch syndrome (LS) is a common hereditary colorectal cancer (CRC) syndrome, diagnosis of LS in daily clinical practice is still difficult due to the insignificant manifestation of the disease compared to other hereditary CRCs such as FAP, which typically develops thousands of polyps in a large intestine simply identified by colonoscopy. Assembly of CRCs in patients within a family was first published by Bashford in 1908 [1]. However, he thought that the disease comes from environmental factor but not from heredity.

Concept of LS was initially recognized by a pathologist and physician Aldred S. Warthin at the University of Michigan in 1913, who carefully listened to one of his patients, seamstress, and gathered an extensive family history and proposed a familial explanation for this phenomenon [2].

Of course, Dr. Warthin followed up his own family members, Henry T. Lynch and others also intensively followed his work, finally finding numerous similar families in a variety of communities and countries [3–5].

The investigators recognized that some familial CRCs were associated with a novel cancer "pathway," replication error (RER), or microsatellite instability (MSI), that had been independently discovered by two groups who did not suspect that there might be a familial form of this pathway [6–8]. The identification of thoroughly defined families led to the linkage of the cancer-prone phenotype to a single locus of chromosome 2p in 1993 [9]. Then, the discovery of one of the causative gene (*MSH2*) of Lynch syndrome was made in 1994 [10]. A focused race finally led to the discovery of the four genes, *MSH2*, *MLH1*, *PMS2*, and *MSH6*, responsible for LS [11].

Informed by the knowledge of genetic basis of the disease, that driven by the development and validation of two powerful clinical tools, MSI and immunohistochemistry (IH), which allowed progress in the diagnosis and treatment of LS. Now almost all LS cases can be diagnosed by the universal screening for developed CRC and other related cancers, which means that all indicate cases of CRC should be screened by MSI or IH and then sequencing for the responsible four genes if necessary [12].

However, more than 20 years have passed since the discovery of the responsible genes for LS, still full picture of the disease is unclear because of the nature of rare diseases, which strongly suggests the importance of international collaborations.

13.2 History of International Collaboration Group for LS from ICG-HNPCC to InSiGHT

The international collaboration group for LS was established as an ICG-HNPCC (International collaborative group on hereditary non-polyposis colorectal cancer). During the second International Conference on Gastrointestinal Cancer organized by Paul Rosen in Jerusalem in August 1989, Giuseppe Cristofaro from Italy, proposed to Henry T. Lynch that they should form a group of interested colleagues throughout the world to study LS (hereditary non-polyposis colorectal cancer: HNPCC at that time) and to form multiple collaborations in the interest of investigating the genetic, clinical, and pathologic aspects of the disease. Then, Henry T. Lynch, Jane Lynch, Patrick Lynch, Jukka-Pekka Mecklin, Giuseppe Cristofaro, Jim St. John, and Hans Vasen met informally and agreed that this idea was quite reasonable because of the growing interest in LS.

The study of large numbers of families with detailed pedigrees would be required given the syndrome's genotypic and phenotypic heterogeneity. Careful clinical histories, molecular genetics, pathology, surveillance, and management concerns as well as genetic counseling are needed for better understanding of the disease. Of courese benefit for the high-risk patients and their families was be most important issue in ICG-HNPCC. Further discussion about the establishment of the ICG-HNPCC took place in November 1989 at an International Meeting on Colorectal Cancer sponsored by Joji Utsunomiya in Kobe, Japan.

The ICG-HNPCC council initially thought that it might be best to keep the group to a maximum of about 50 members. However, interest in LS around the world was increasing proportionately to numerous publications appearing on the subject of LS and the discovery of the existence and function of the DNA mismatch repair genes. Membership in the group has since been unrestricted and has reflected the broad range of specialties involved in the scientific and clinical aspects of LS.

Following are how the ICG-HNPCC then International Society for Gastrointestinal Hereditary Tumors (InSiGHT) has taken place until recently.

In 1990, Hans Vasen organized the first formal meeting of ICG-HNPCC in Amsterdam, the Netherlands. Thirty representatives from eight countries were present, and a report of this meeting was published in Diseases of Colon and Rectum [13]. It was at that time that the first Amsterdam criteria for a clinical diagnosis of HNPCC based on family history were established [14]. Publication of amended Amsterdam Criteria allowing inclusion and extracolonic cancers in the clinical definition of HNPCC (LS) (Table 13.1).

13.3 International Collaborative Groups Related to InSiGHT

13.3.1 The InSiGHT Database: LOVD System

InSiGHT operates database with sharing of clinical and genetic variant data for genes associated with inherited CRCs. The Leiden Open Variation Database (LOVD) technology used for this task has been updated to handle genomic data that is increasingly being generated. InSiGHT maintains a database of known mutations in the mismatch repair genes [15]. This has been of great usefulness in determining the significance of mutations as they are reported. The governance committee (Drs Peltomaki, Woods, Sijmons, Vasem, dem Dummem, and Macrae) met early in the year to guide the progress of the InSiGHT databases [16].

Table 13.1 History of International Collaborative Group on Hereditary Non-Polyposis Colorectal Cancer (ICG-HNPCC) to International Society for Gastrointestinal Hereditary Tumors (InSiGHT)

1991	Trino, Italy ICG-HNPCC meeting organized by Giuseppe Cristofaro
1992	Crete, Greece ICG-HNPCC meeting organized by Hans Vasen
1993	Houston, USA ICG-HNPCC meeting organized by Patrick Lynch
1994	Milan, Italy, organized ICG-HNPCC meeting by Lucio Bertario
1995	Helsinki, Finland ICG-HNPCC meeting organized by J.P. Mecklin
1996	Buffalo, New York, USA ICG-HNPCC meeting organized by Miguel Rodriguez-Bigas
1997	Noordwijk, The Netherlands 1st combined meeting of ICG-HNPCC with the Leeds Castle Polyposis Group (LCPG) by Hans Vasen
1998	Coimbra, Portugal ICG-HNPCC meeting by Julio Leite
1999	Lorne/Melbourne, Australia Second combined meeting of ICG-HNPCC and LCPG, organized by Finlay Macrae
2000	Tiberias, Israel ICG-HNPCC meeting organized by Paul Rosen
2001	Venice, Italy Third combined meeting of ICG-HNPCC and LCPG, organized by Lucio Bertario.
2003	Cleveland, Ohio, USA Fourth combined meeting of LCPG and ICG-HNPCC organized by James Church LCPG and ICG-HNPCC merged to InSiGHT
2005	NewCastle, UK First conference of InSiGHT organized by Sir John Burn
2007	Yokohama, Japan Second conference of InSiGHT by Takeo Iwama
2009	Dusseldorf, Germany Third conference of InSiGHT by Gabriela Moslein
2011	San Antonio, Texas, USA Fourth conference of InSiGHT by Patrick Lynch and Miguel Rodoriguez Bigas
2013	Cairns, Australia Fifth conference of InSiGHT by Allan Spigelman
2015	Sao Paulo, Brazil Sixth conference of InSiGHT by Benedio Rossi
2017	Florence, Italy Seventh conference of InSiGHT by Maurizio Genuardi and Luigi Ricciardiello
2019	Auckland, New Zealand Eighth conference of InSiGHT by Susan Parry

There has been an exciting activity around the mismatch repair database [17]. Firstly, there are continuing efforts to encourage submissions of variant data to the database. It is obviously clear that all genes need good locus-specific databases so as to support the activities of health professionals caring for families with genetic diseases. The InSiGHT database receives 20,000 hits/month for information to aid in interpretation. Its value is only as good as the comprehensiveness of its submissions.

The database also adds value. Maurizio Genuardi chairs an Interpretation Committee of over 45 of our colleagues who are systematically addressing all the information around all unclassified variants on the database and reaching an assessment of the pathogenicity based on all published and unpublished information available [18].

13.3.2 InSiGHT and the Human Variome Project

InSiGHT is cooperating closely with the Human Variome Project and has become its first gene-specific member [19]. InSiGHT is represented on the HVP Scientific Advisory Committee. The processes and procedures InSiGHT has developed to support its databases have been acclaimed by the HVP as a leading model and are being replicated across many genes. InSiGHT benefits from the broad experience of members of the HVP, with their expertise in locus-specific databases, ethical considerations, international reach, and, most importantly, recognition by UNESCO.

13.3.3 Other InSiGHT Database Collaborations

The success of the database and its processes has attracted interest from several stakeholders in the HVP to draw on its experience and outcomes. Amongst these has been an inclusion in an NIH application to support the flow of data (MutaDatabase) from the US private diagnostic labs to the National Center for Biotechnology Information (NCBI) (Clin Var), access to the deliberations of the Interpretation Committee to test a new data model (PathoDB) being developed in the EU's Gen2Phen project, and models of interchange with the UK Diagnostic Services' central database (DMuDB) and French national database. Direct negotiations with Quest Diagnostics, the largest private US lab, are also in place. Incorporation has assisted in all these areas.

13.3.4 Collaborative Group of the Americans on Inherited Colorectal Cancer (CGA-ICC) to CGA-IG(Gastrointestinal)C

The Collaborative Group of the Americans on Inherited Colorectal Cancer (CGA-ICC) was established in 1995 to improve understanding of the basic science of inherited colorectal cancer and the clinical management of affected families [20]. In 2018, the CGA-ICC moved to change their name to the Collaborative Group of the Americans on Inherited Gastrointestinal Cancer (CGA-IGC), to be more inclusive of inherited gastrointestinal cancers as a whole. The CGA-IGC's clinical and research focus is hereditary gastrointestinal cancers syndromes, including but not limited to: Familial adenomatous polyposis (FAP), MUTYH associated polyposis (MAP), Polymerase proofreading-associated polyposis (PPAP), Peutz-Jeghers syndrome, PTEN tumor-hamartoma syndrome, Hereditary mixed polyposis syndrome, Lynch syndrome, Familial colorectal cancer type X, and Hyperplastic polyposis/serrated polyposis. The vision of the CGA-IGC is to eliminate morbidity and mortality of hereditary gastrointestinal cancers. The mission of the CGA-IGC is to advance science of inherited gastrointestinal cancers through research and education as the leading authority in the Americans. Through this mission, the CGA-ICG offers the following:

- Education regarding the clinical management and molecular genetics of inherited gastrointestinal cancer to physicians, allied healthcare professionals, patients, and their families
- Access to collaborative trials and studies
- Resources for developing new hereditary registries and supporting their registries
- A forum for exchange of ideas
- Multidisciplinary expertise in clinical care, healthcare policy and research related to hereditary gastrointestinal cancer

13.3.5 European Hereditary Tumor Group (EHTG)

European Hereditary Tumor Group (EHTG) was devolved from the former "Mallorca Group." The Mallorca Group was initiated in 2006 by Hans Vasen and Gabriela Moeslein and was a very active network of specialists working in different fields involved with prevention, diagnosis, and treatment of hereditary tumor syndromes. The focus was laid on gastrointestinal predisposition to tumors but may now evolve to embrace other.

The group has defined the aims as:

- To conduct collaborative studies
- To establish guidelines
- To set up databases

The working group format as a most interactive platform was most well received during the first meeting of the EHTG in Mallorca in 2016.

In 2017, EHTG supported the InSiGHT meeting in Florence and hosted a 1-day meeting on July 5.

In 2018, the third meeting of the EHTG took place on September 23–25, 2008 in Nice, France with connected with ESCP. Joint EHTG/ESCP symposium at ESCP on Wednesday September 26.

Fourth meeting of EHTG was held in Barcelona, Spain on October 17–19 ahead of UEG Week.

- PLSD: The Prospective Lynch Syndrome Database: Pal Moller
- Guidelines for Juvenile Polyposis: Karli Heinimann

- Guidelines for MAP, PPAP, and NAP: Julian Sampson and Stefan Aretz
- European Database C4CMMRD: Chrystelle Colas
- De novo MMR mutations in Lynch Syndrome: Ian Frying
- New Juvenile Polyposis Genes: Ian Tomlinson
- Identification of predictors of CRC development in MMR mutation carriers under colonoscopy surveillance: Francesc Balaguer
- Role of Genetic Modifiers in Disease Risk-Lynch Syndrome: Bente Talseth-Palmer

13.3.6 PLSD (the Prospective Lynch Syndrome Database)

LS is associated with a high probability of GI, gynecological, and other cancers. It is caused by inherited mutations affecting any of four DNA mismatch repair (MMR) genes, *MSH2*, *MLH1*, *PMS2*, or *MSH6*, or by a deletion in the *EPCAM* gene, which leads to methylation of the adjacent *MSH2* promoter. It is an under-recognized condition accounting for about 1–3% of colorectal cancers in the population. To date, most LS patients have been identified following investigation because of their family or personal histories of multiple and/or early-onset cancers.

Carriers of pathogenic *MLH1*, *MSH2*, *MSH6*, or *PMS2* mutations requite reliable information about their future cancer risk so that they can be offered appropriately targeted surveillance, but published risk estimates are extremely variable. One obvious factor is reliance on retrospective data. Another is the impact of initial selection criteria for molecular testing. In clinical practice, these have included the Amsterdam I or Amsterdam II criteria, the Bethesda guidelines or simply age at cancer diagnosis. Previous estimates of the cumulative risk at 70 years for CRC in *MLH1* or *MSH2* mutation carriers range from 22 to 74%. Mutation of *MSH6* or *PMS2* genes have lower penetrance and different patterns of expression: *MSH6* mutation carriers are thought to have a high risk of endometrial cancer, similar to that in *MSH2* mutation carriers, but lower risks of CRC. For a comprehensive and updated overview or literature, see two recently published reviews by us an others. Colonoscopy enables the identification and removal of preinvasive neoplasia or early cancers in the absence of symptoms and is the mainstay of secondary prevention in LS patients. Although adenoma removal is considered to represent a surrogate for the prevention of CRC and death, the evidence supporting this assumption in LS is controversial.

EHTG have developed a pooled prospective database of LS mutation carriers to better characterize their cancer risks and the effects of interventions [21–23].

Objectives include:

1. Prospective observations in carriers of pathogenic variants causing Lynch syndrome
2. Report prospectively observed events by observation years
3. Categorizing observations by gene, gender, age, and intervention(s)
4. Result publicly available through open access publications

5. Results publicly available as an interactive website to calculate cancer risk for any given carrier of pathogenic variant causing LS
6. Through the above arrive on empirically obtained knowledge as basis for
   - Scientific studies
   - Guidance for health care

13.3.7 International Mismatch Repair Consortium (IMRC)

To bridge critical gaps in LS research, the International Mismatch Repair Consortium (IMRC) was formed in 2010. The IMRC comprises major worldwide consortiums involved in the research and/or clinical treatment of LS (cancer predisposition caused by inherited mutations in mismatch repair (MMR) genes: *MLH1*, *MSH2*, *MSH6*, *PMS2*, and *EPCAM*); http://www.sphinx.org.au/imrc.

The establishment of the IMRC was facilitated by the InSiGHT and the CGA-ICC. Currently, the IMRC has 205 members from 74 centers/clinics in Africa, Australasia, Europe, North America, and South America, and membership is open to anyone involved in research related to LS and/or the treatment of LS families. Recently Japan also joined the consortium by submitting our small data. Accurate cancer risk estimates are needed to develop genetic counseling guidelines and are of importance for the clinical management of mutation carriers and members within high-risk families. Risk may differ not only by age and gender and the gene that is mutated but also by the country and ethnicity of the carrier. The only way to thoroughly address this potential heterogeneity is to conduct comprehensive penetrance analysis on large, ethnically heterogeneous samples of persons/families segregating mutations in MMR genes.

Aim of the IMRC:

- Establish a combined data set of pedigree data from around the world for approximately 8800 Lynch syndrome families.
- Estimate the age-specific cumulative risk (penetrance) of cancers at each anatomical site by sex, mismatch repair gene, type of mutation, and nationality/geographic region.
- Develop a personal risk tool for clinical use that provides 10-years risks of cancer based on the age, sex, mismatch repair gen, type of mutation, and nationality/geographic region.

Since July 2014, IMRC investigators from 63 sites were contacted and requested to submit the MMR family data from their clinics/centers. Instructions on the preferred data format were provided, including data dictionaries for personal and family history of demographic data, cancer, MMR gene mutation status, screening, surgery, and mortality. April 2016, 28 investigators representing 38 sites of 18 countries have submitted MMR pedigree data for 4302 families including 11,418 mutation carriers.

Collection of MMR family data from many international sites, with varying resources (Many of which were not established or designed for epidemiological research), is challenging. The IMRC will be investigating ways to facilitate data collection for this project to ensure the maximum benefit is gained from this collegial and international consortium.

13.3.8 Cancer Prevention Project 3 (CAPP3)

The aim of this study is to find the right dose of aspirin for chemoprevention in LS. The Cancer Prevention Project 3 (CAPP3) study is endorsed by InSiGHT. Over 100 epidemiological/observational studies have reported a significant reduction in cancer among long-term regular users of aspirin and other nonsteroidal anti-inflammatory drugs (NSAIDS). Meta-analysis of randomized controlled trials using colonic adenomas as an endpoint has revealed a significant reduction in that given aspirin. Very long-term follow-up of participants in early cardiovascular trials revealed a 21% reduction in cancer mortality among those randomized to the aspirin limbs, commencing from 5 years after randomization. Two randomized control trials with cancer as a primary endpoint have now reported a significant effect:

- CAPP2 randomized 1009 carriers of hereditary colorectal cancer (LS due to mutation in mismatch repair gene) to 600 mg aspirin daily for up to 4 years [24]. Those who complied with the primary aim of treatment for at least 2 years saw a 63% reduction in colorectal cancer and comparable reduction in other cancers associated with the syndrome such as endometrial cancer. The effects become apparent from 4 years from 4 years after commencing the trial.
- The Women's Health Study gave alternate day 100 mg aspirin for 10 years to 10,000 American women. There was no effect on cancer at the trial end but subsequent follow-up has revealed an 18% reduction in CRC with the effect becoming apparent after 10 years [25].

There is an expert consensus that aspirin should be recommended to those at high risk but ongoing debate about the optimal dose and the risk benefit ratio in the general population. CAPP3 will test three different doses 600, 300, and 100 mg enteric-coated aspirin in 3000 mismatch repair gene defect carriers at risk of LS. All 3000 participants will be receiving aspirin until the end of the study. Results are expected in 2020. Meanwhile, low dose aspirin can be recommended to any high-risk individuals not taking part in the trial.

13.4 Conclusions

International collaboration in LS was crucial and basis for recognition, understanding, and treatment of this rare disease (syndrome). Mainstream of the international collaboration was undertaken through ICG-HNPCC and then InSiGHT. Important branch of collaborations related to these mainstream collaborations are also listed.

References

1. Bashford. Discussion on the influence of heredity on disease, with special reference to tuberculosis, cancer, and diseases of the nervous system: introductory address. Proc R Soc Med. 1909;(2(Gen Rep)):63–75.
2. Warthin AS. Hereditary with reference to carcinoma. Arch Intern Med (Chic). 1913;12:546–55.
3. Warthin AS. The further study of a cancer family. J Cancer Res. 1925;9:278–86.
4. Hauser JJ, Weller CV. A further report on the cancer family of Warthin. Am J Cancer. 1936;27:454–44.
5. Lynch HT, Krush AJ. Cancer family "G" revisited: 1895–1970. Cancer. 1971;27(6):1505–11.
6. Ionov Y, Peinado MA, Malkhosyan S, Shibata D, Perucho M. Ubiquitous somatic mutations in simple repeated sequences reveal a new mechanism for colonic carcinogenesis. Nature. 1993;363(6429):558–61.
7. Thibodeau SN, Bren G, Schaid D. Microsatellite instability in cancer of the proximal colon. Science. 1993;260(5109):816–9.
8. Aaltonen LA, Peltomaki P, Leach FS, et al. Clues to the pathogenesis of familial colorectal cancer. Science. 1993;260(5109):812–6.
9. Peltomaki P, Aaltonen LA, Sistonen P, et al. Genetic mapping of a locus predisposing to human colorectal cancer. Science. 1993;260(5109):810–2.
10. Fishel R, Lescoe MK, Rao MR, et al. The human mutator gene homolog MSH2 and its association with hereditary nonpolyposis colon cancer. Cell. 1994;77(1):1 p following 166.
11. Bronner CE, Baker SM, Morrison PT, et al. Mutation in the DNA mismatch repair gene homologue hMLH1 is associated with hereditary non-polyposis colon cancer. Nature. 1994;368(6468):258–61.
12. Perez-Carbonell L, Ruiz-Ponte C, Guarinos C, et al. Comparison between universal molecular screening for Lynch syndrome and revised Bethesda guidelines in a large population-based cohort of patients with colorectal cancer. Gut. 2012;61(6):865–72.
13. Vasen HF, Mecklin JP, Watson P, et al. Surveillance in hereditary nonpolyposis colorectal cancer: an international cooperative study of 165 families. The International Collaborative Group on HNPCC. Dis Colon Rectum. 1993;36(1):1–4.
14. Vasen HF, Mecklin JP, Khan PM, Lynch HT. The International Collaborative Group on Hereditary Non-Polyposis Colorectal Cancer (ICG-HNPCC). Dis Colon Rectum. 1991;34(5):424–5.
15. Fokkema IF, Taschner PE, Schaafsma GC, Celli J, Laros JF, den Dunnen JT. LOVD v.2.0: the next generation in gene variant databases. Hum Mutat. 2011;32(5):557–63.
16. Peltomaki P, Vasen HF. Mutations predisposing to hereditary nonpolyposis colorectal cancer: database and results of a collaborative study. The International Collaborative Group on Hereditary Nonpolyposis Colorectal Cancer. Gastroenterology. 1997;113(4):1146–58.
17. Plazzer JP, Sijmons RH, Woods MO, et al. The InSiGHT database: utilizing 100 years of insights into Lynch syndrome. Familial Cancer. 2013;12(2):175–80.
18. Sijmons RH, Greenblatt MS, Genuardi M. Gene variants of unknown clinical significance in Lynch syndrome. An introduction for clinicians. Familial Cancer. 2013;12(2):181–7.
19. Kaput J, Cotton RG, Hardman L, et al. Planning the human variome project: the Spain report. Hum Mutat. 2009;30(4):496–510.
20. Weissman SM, Burt R, Church J, et al. Identification of individuals at risk for Lynch syndrome using targeted evaluations and genetic testing: National Society of Genetic Counselors and the Collaborative Group of the Americas on Inherited Colorectal Cancer joint practice guideline. J Genet Couns. 2012;21(4):484–93.
21. Moller P, Seppala T, Bernstein I, et al. Cancer incidence and survival in Lynch syndrome patients receiving colonoscopic and gynaecological surveillance: first report from the prospective Lynch syndrome database. Gut. 2017;66(3):464–72.

22. Moller P, Seppala T, Bernstein I, et al. Incidence of and survival after subsequent cancers in carriers of pathogenic MMR variants with previous cancer: a report from the prospective Lynch syndrome database. Gut. 2017;66(9):1657–64.
23. Moller P, Seppala TT, Bernstein I, et al. Cancer risk and survival in path_MMR carriers by gene and gender up to 75 years of age: a report from the Prospective Lynch Syndrome Database. Gut. 2018;67(7):1306–16.
24. Burn J, Gerdes AM, Macrae F, et al. Long-term effect of aspirin on cancer risk in carriers of hereditary colorectal cancer: an analysis from the CAPP2 randomised controlled trial. Lancet. 2011;378(9809):2081–7.
25. Ait Ouakrim D, Dashti SG, Chau R, et al. Aspirin, ibuprofen, and the risk of colorectal cancer in Lynch syndrome. J Natl Cancer Inst. 2015;107(9):djv170.

MIX
Papier aus verantwortungsvollen Quellen
Paper from responsible sources
FSC® C105338

If you have any concerns about our products,
you can contact us on
ProductSafety@springernature.com

In case Publisher is established outside the EU,
the EU authorized representative is:
Springer Nature Customer Service Center GmbH
Europaplatz 3, 69115 Heidelberg, Germany

Printed by Libri Plureos GmbH
in Hamburg, Germany